BEAST BOWL NUTRITION

100+ MAKE-AHEAD AND MAKE NOW MEAL-PREP RECIPES THE WHOLE FAMILY WILL LOVE

FOODOLOGY GEEK

LAURA REIGEL

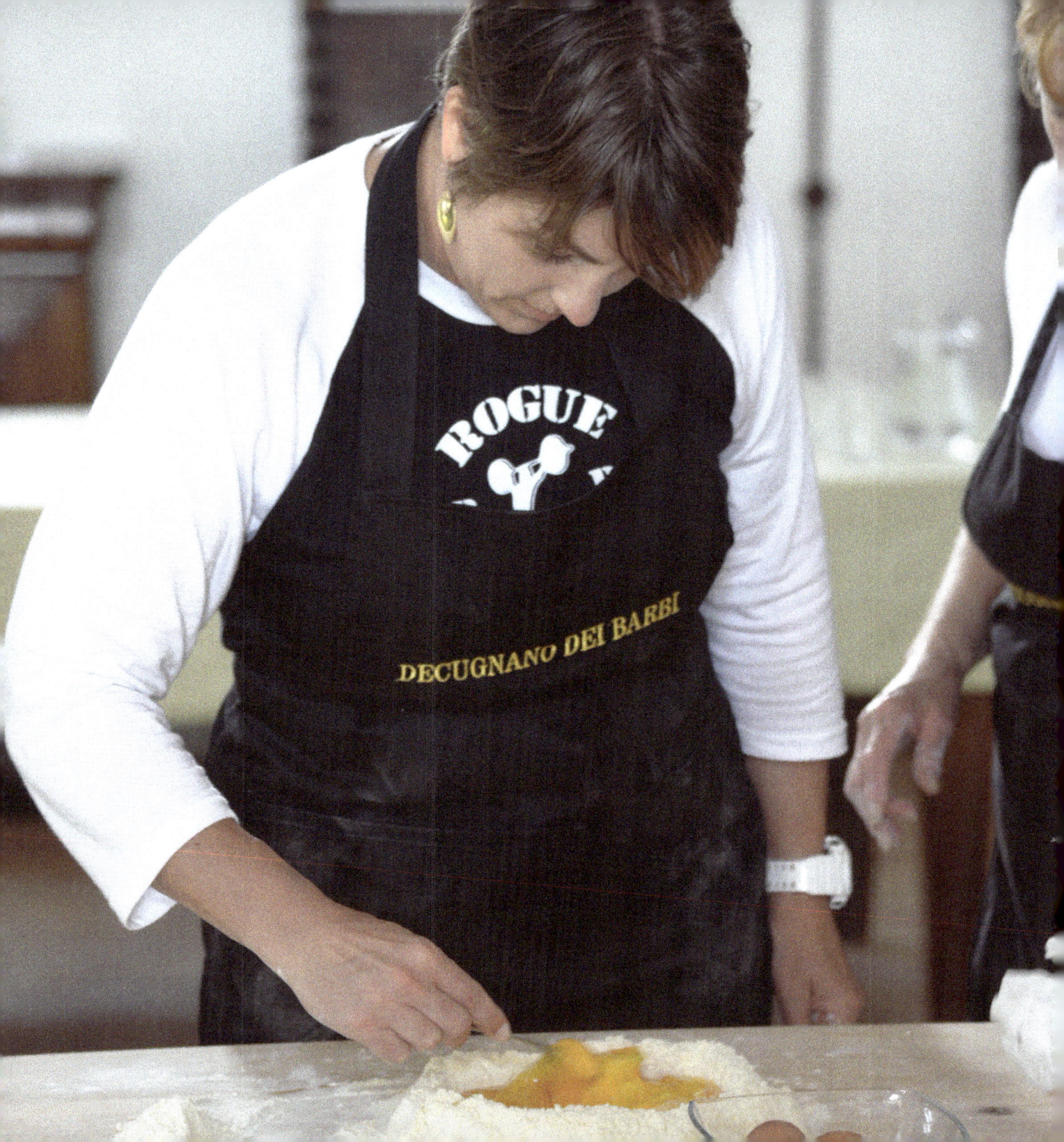

BEAST BOWL NUTRITION IS BUILT FOR FITNESS-MINDED FOODIES

Eating real food for real is the most sustainable way to stay healthy. This cookbook gives you beautifully designed whole food recipes that you will want to eat! All of the recipes in this cookbook are designed to have NO gluten, NO dairy, and NO refined sugar, except for the occasional, completely optional sprinkle of cheese. Plus they're all designed to be vegan adaptable. Feed everyone in your family healthy and easy to prepare meals.

Visit me at FoodologyGeek.com to find out more!

FOODOLOGY GEEK
Real Food · For Real

This cookbook was written with love in conjunction with FoodologyGeek.com

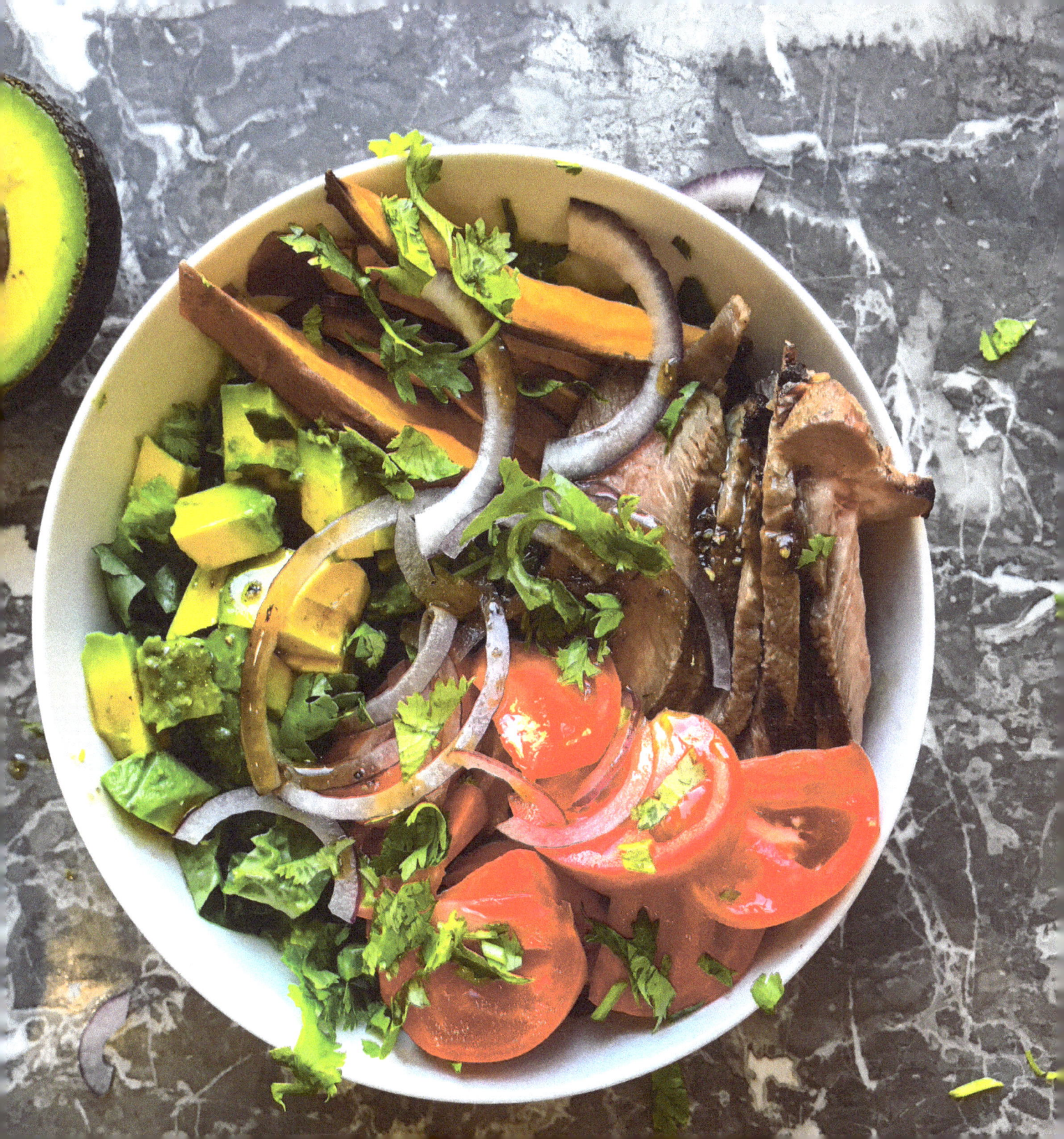

©2019 Foodology Geek and Beast Bowl Nutrition

All rights reserved. This book or any portion thereof may not be reproduced or used in any manner whatsoever without the express written permission of the publisher except for the use of brief quotations in a book review.

The scanning, uploading, and distribution of this book without permission is a theft of the author's intellectual property. If you would like permission to use material from the book (other than for review purposes), please contact cookbook@foodologygeek.com. Thank you for your support of the author's rights.

Published in the United States of America

First Edition: 2019

ISBN 978-1-7329059-2-4

Foodology Geek
4750-124 Almaden Expressway, PMB 385
San Jose, CA 95118
FoodologyGeek.com

Editorial Director: Laura Reigel
Editor: Karie Stephens
Photography and Logo Design: Laura Reigel
Recipe Creator: Laura Reigel

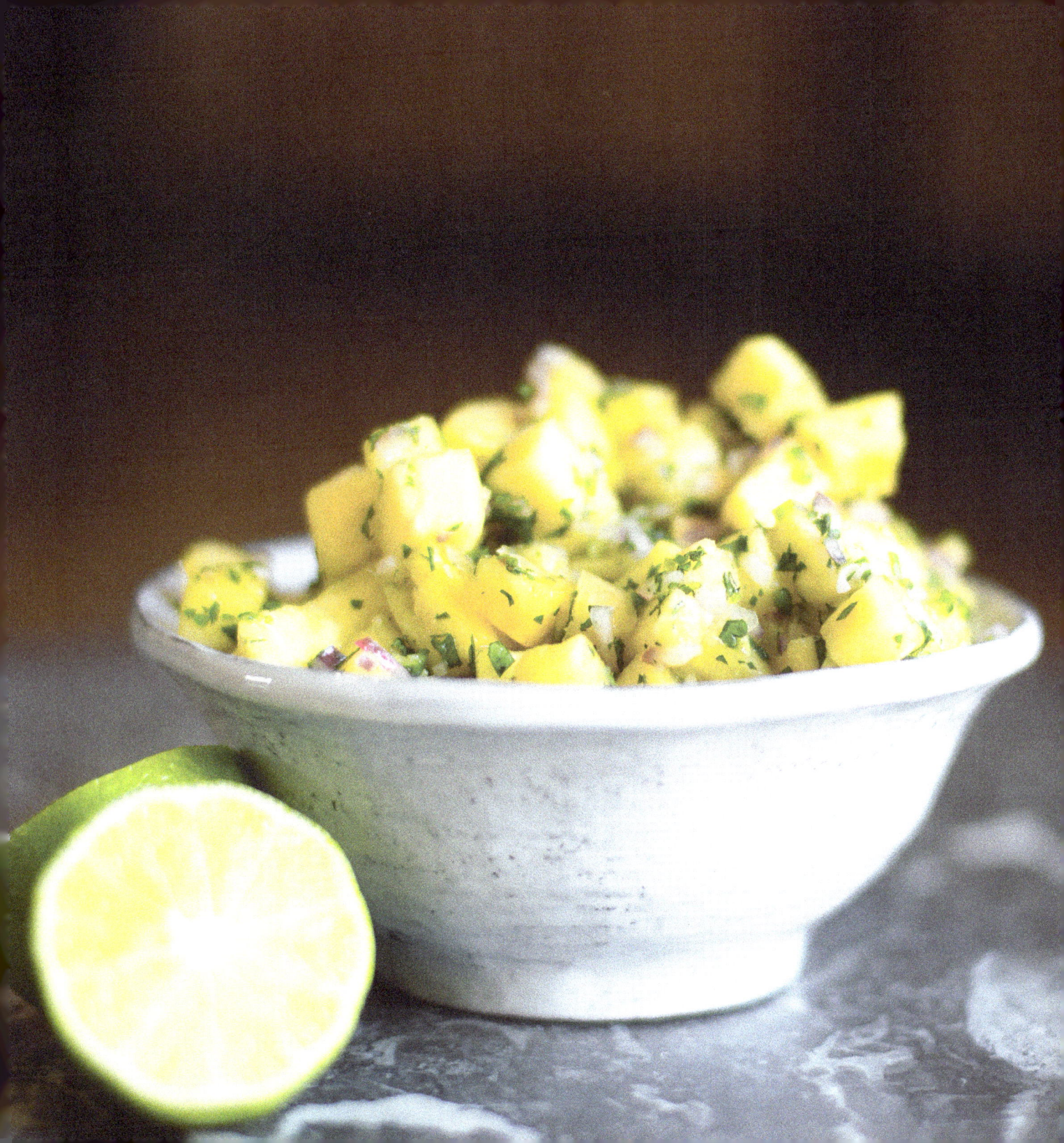

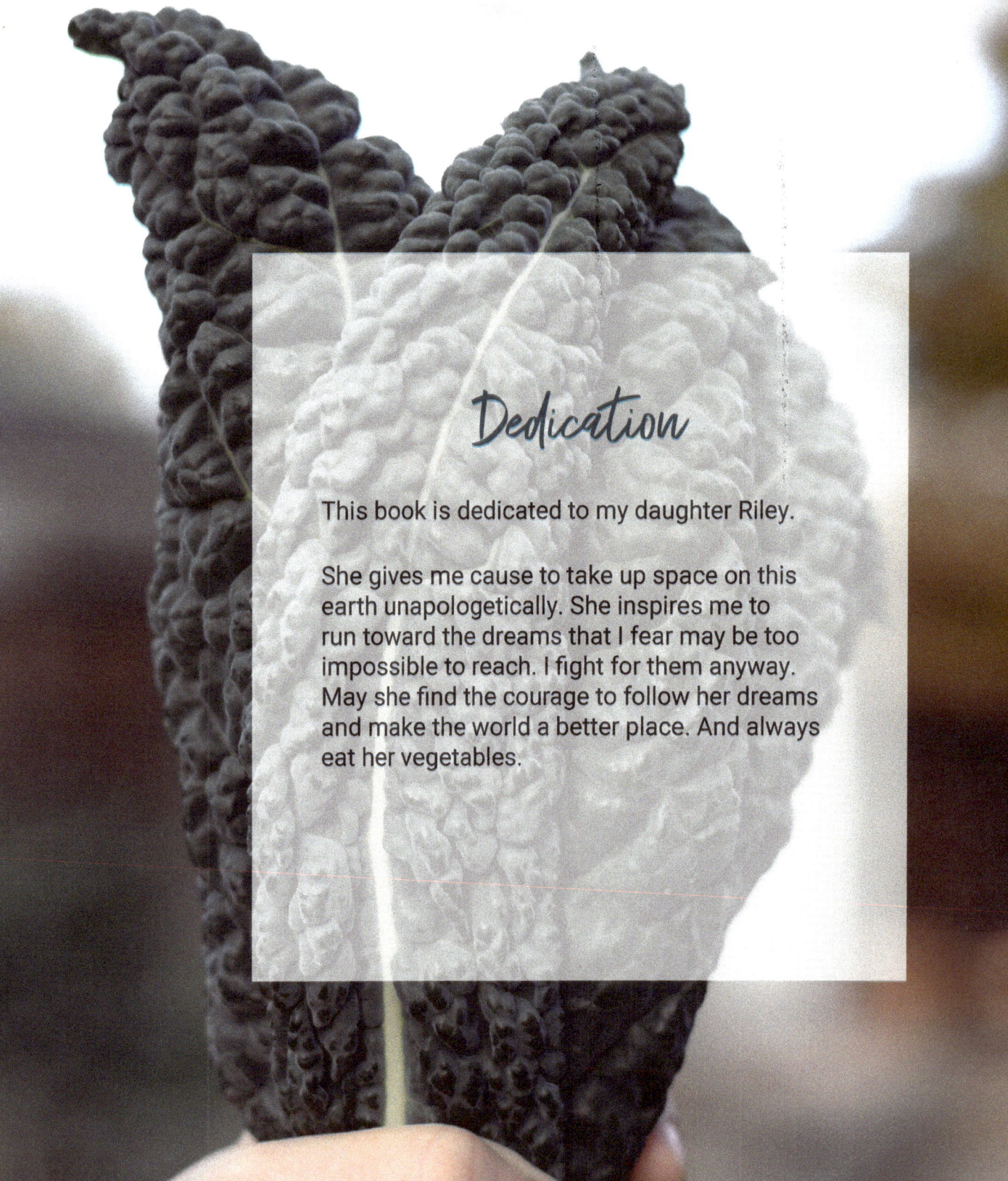

Dedication

This book is dedicated to my daughter Riley.

She gives me cause to take up space on this earth unapologetically. She inspires me to run toward the dreams that I fear may be too impossible to reach. I fight for them anyway. May she find the courage to follow her dreams and make the world a better place. And always eat her vegetables.

TABLE OF CONTENTS

Foreword	**1**
The Concept	**4**
Building A Bowl	**16**
Meal Prep 101	**31**
Core Proteins & Extras	**40**
Paleo Breakfast	43
Breakfast Hash	45
Asian Chicken Meatball	47
Asian Cucumber Salad	49
Asian Dressing	49
Asian Slaw	51
Asian Peanut Slaw Dressing	51
Lemongrass Shrimp	53
Pickled Asian Veggies	55
Teriyaki Chicken	57
⚒ How To Meal Prep In 5 Minutes	**59**
Chicken Satay	61
⚒ The Right Tools Make It Easy	**63**
Chili Verde	65
Mexican Guacamole	67
Chipotle Chicken	69

Roasted Corn Salsa	71
Salsa Fresca	72
Tequila Lime Fish	**75**
Mango Salsa	77
Barbecue Pulled Pork	**79**
Southern Coleslaw	80
Coleslaw Dressing	80
Fried Chicken	**83**
⚒ The Science Of Fat	**85**
Buffalo Chicken	**87**
All-American Burger	**89**
Steak Chimichurri	**93**
Tostones	95
Columbian Guacamole	97
Mom-Style Taco	**99**
Mexican Slaw	101
Provençal Chicken & Veggies	**103**
Blanched Green Beans	105
Jamaican Jerk Chicken	**107**
Roasted Plantains	109
Pineapple Salsa	110
Jamaican Rice & Peas	113
Greek Lamb Burger	**115**
⚒ Meet Meat	**117**
Paleo Meatloaf	**119**
Cauliflower Smash	121

Mediterranean Fish	123
Shrimp Louie	125
Steak & Sweet Potato	127
Oven Roasted Potatoes	129
Sweet Potato Fries	131
Chicken Lettuce Wraps	133
Carrot & Apple Slaw	135

Dressings & Sauces — 136

✗ Basics of Vinaigrettes	138
Vietnamese Vinaigrette	140
Champagne Vinaigrette	142
Citrus Vinaigrette	142
Greek Vinaigrette	144
Herbes de Provence Vinaigrette	144
Mustard Vinaigrette	145
Red Wine Vinaigrette	145
Sesame Ginger Vinaigrette	147
Tomato Balsamic Vinaigrette	147
✗ Basics of Mayo	148
Beastastic Mayo	153
Paleo Ranch	155
Buffalo Ranch	156
Chipotle Ranch	157
Beast Sauce	158
Louie Dressing	158
Garlicky Aioli	159

Remoulade	159
Avocado Cilantro Lime Crema	161
Chipotle Crema	163
Chimichurri Sauce	165
Paleo Ketchup	167
Tzatziki	169
Lemon Tahini Dressing	171
Spicy Tangy Barbecue Sauce	173
Peach Bourbon Barbecue Sauce	175
Onion Jam	177
Spicy Tomato Jam	179
Satay Peanut Sauce	181

Seasonings 183

Mediterranean	185
Herbes de Provence	185
Buffalo	186
Pumpkin Pie Spice	186
Barbecue Rub	187
Jamaican Jerk	187
Taco	188

Snacks 189

Almond Bark	193
Chai Latte Chia Pudding	195
Chocolate Chia Pudding	197
Strawberry Chia Pudding	199

Rocky Road Fudge	201
Hazelnut Chocolate Chip Cookies	203
Paleo Granola Bites	205
Strawberry Mojito Nice Cream	207
Savory Roasted Nuts	209

What To Make Tonight? — 210

Got Chicken?	212
Got Beef?	212
Got Pork?	212
Got Seafood?	212
Core Proteins	213
Plant-Based	213

Acknowledgements — 214

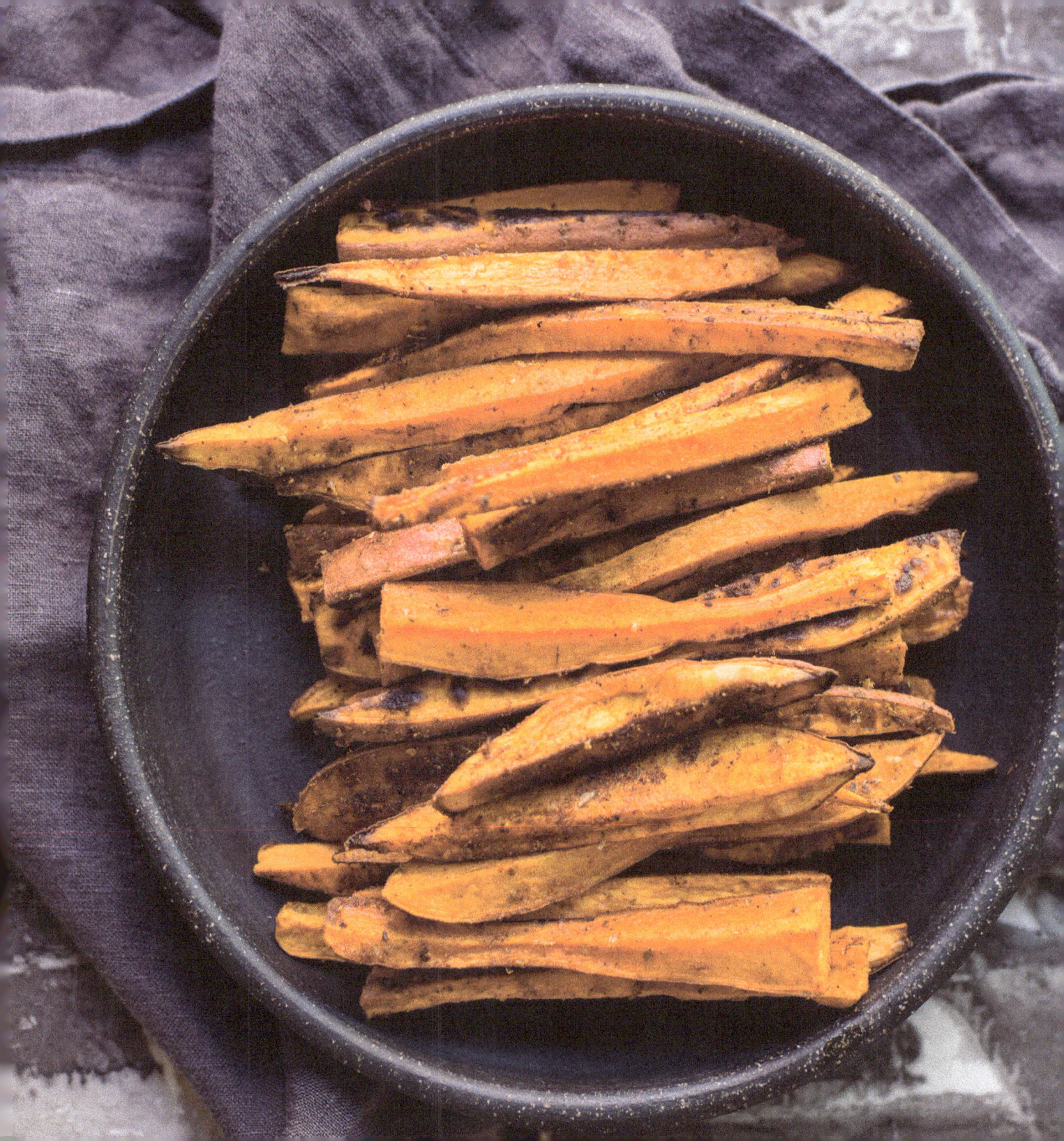

Foreword

I've long been inspired by science — physiology, biochemistry, and metabolic biochemistry. I studied physiology and neuroscience in college, and, eventually, forensic science. I ended up using my love of science to investigate crime as a DNA analyst, crime scene investigator, and cold case homicide investigator… but that's a story for another day.

My passions for science and for cooking have blended perfectly in the study of nutrition. I am a longtime athlete, so healthy eating has always been part of my life. My experience studying nutrition and coaching clients was the biggest driver for writing this book. Planning healthy food takes effort and practice. The struggle is real! We are all busy, and living with people who may not be as ambitious about healthy eating can lead to major frustration. A lot of times it can end up pushing you down that path of just picking up the phone and ordering a deep dish. Don't do that! Make a Beast Bowl instead.

I started my blog, *Foodology Geek,* to explore my interest in cooking, photography, and delicious recipes. This blog space is my creative outlet, and now I get to use my crime scene photography skills on a much more pleasant subject matter: beautiful and delicious food.

After about a year of blogging, a clear trend started to surface. The food that I enjoyed cooking and eating most of the time usually comprised a core protein, a lot of veggies, and some type of dressing or sauce. My readers also wanted to see more of this kind of cooking. Perfect for meal prep! I'm a busy working mom, so I needed recipes that aren't super time consuming, but because I'm a hardcore foodie, I also needed recipes that taste delicious.

I wrote *Beast Bowl Nutrition* as a resource that includes sustainable, nutritious, and delicious meal ideas for you and your family. I know how hard it can be to get dinner on the table every night, let alone a healthy dinner! Cooking for a family can be tricky. When I wrote this book, my daughter had been vegan for over two years. My husband is a committed meat-and-potatoes kind of guy. And I'm an omnivorous food snob who likes to eat real food that tastes amazing. I needed recipes that would satisfy all of us.

This book is also good for people who are cooking for a family member that might have different dietary restrictions. Almost every recipe includes notes about making the recipes gluten-free, dairy-free, and/or vegan. Many of my best friends have food allergies, some of them are following keto diets, and some of them are just picky eaters. These recipes are for them, too.

I started cooking Beast Bowl-style during my nutrition coaching program because I realized that I wasn't getting enough fresh vegetables in my diet. I've always loved protein and thought I ate enough veggies, but when I really started taking a look at it, I realized I was only eating broccoli and green beans. No wonder I was bored as heck with my meal planning!

For all the fitness-minded foodies out there who want to stay lean but actually have a palate, *Beast Bowl Nutrition* was written for you. You want to eat food that fuels your training, keeps you lean, and doesn't taste like soggy, microwaved broccoli and flavorless, bland baked chicken breasts.

I hope you enjoy all of the Beast Bowls in this book. I hope you will find some inspiration to cook a little more. And most importantly, I hope the tools and suggestions in this book make it just a little bit easier to eat healthfully.

Maybe some of these recipes might even help to give you a sense of peace when you are planning weekly meals for you and whomever else you might be cooking for. These recipes will make it easy for you to prep your meals and have healthy food in the fridge all week long.

ONE MORE THING: Every recipe in this book is a suggestion. Please start out with what you can do well. Use prepared dressings until you feel comfortable making your own.

Use the shortcuts any time you need to. No guilt! Time is limited, but we all need to eat, so just do your best. Practice makes perfect!

You can always find me at FoodologyGeek.com/BBN if you need more recipes or real nutrition guidance and coaching. There you'll find everything you need to know about Beast Bowls, meal prep, and nutrition, and of course downloadable tools and resources. I hope to see you there.

CHAPTER 1
THE CONCEPT

Hello Stress-Free Eating

We all know we're supposed to eat healthfully, but come on, you want your food to taste good too. Am I right? Life's just too short to eat microwaved broccoli!

This cookbook will give you a repertoire of healthy go-to recipes that taste amazing and support your fitness and nutrition goals.

Let's get started with the basic concepts behind building a Beast Bowl!

There are four key components to a perfectly planned Beast Bowl. The foremost component, plants, provides colorful micro-nutrition. Then, we have the three macronutrients we all know and love: protein, fat, and carbs.

PLANTS

We've all heard it. Vegetables are important. But how much vegetation do you really need?

Experts recommend ten servings of colorful fruits and vegetables per day. "What? That's ridiculous!" was the first thing that came to my mind when I first heard that. You, too? A serving is approximately equivalent to a large handful, or about one cup.

Most of the recipes in this book were developed for the sole purpose of upping my own plant-eating game. I'm here to help you do the same. Plants show up in two ways when you're eating Beast Bowl-style: the fixins and the extras.

Fixins are the veggies that you might toss into your bowl, such as spinach, shredded carrots, tomatoes, or cucumbers. Fixins also include stuff that isn't in the plant category, but you get the idea. Extras are the sides that go with each bowl. They might include salsa or a slaw, or even something like rice and peas in the Jerk Chicken Beast Bowl!

All of the macro tables can be found at FoodologyGeek.com/BBN – these tables serve as a guide to give you an idea of what each component contributes to the Bowl. I've only included the components that contribute the most significant macro values to each Bowl. Because leafy greens aren't a big deal calorie-wise, I've left them out of the tables. Eat them with reckless abandon.

The Beast Bowl concept assumes that you might put different fixins in your Beast Bowl than I might put in mine. Fixins are the foundation plants, the leafy green and colorful veggie base of the Beast Bowl. This might be lettuce, spinach, carrots, onions... you get the point. These vegetables provide a very important source of micro-nutrition known as phytonutrients. Think of phytonutrients as the building blocks that your metabolism needs to run efficiently.

SUGGESTED FOUNDATION PLANTS (2 TO 3 HANDFULS)

LETTUCES: While iceberg lettuce has its place, try to look outside the box and see all the different lettuce varieties out there. Get out of your comfort zone and try some more flavorful, colorful lettuces.

KALE: There are many varieties of kale. If you've tried one and didn't like it, give another variety a try. Two of my favorites are lacinato kale and baby kale.

SPINACH: Pre-packaged baby spinach is really easy to use. It's great, too, because when you cook it, it reduces down quite a bit. This allows you to get heaping servings of veggies in a lower volume so that you aren't chewing for days.

MICROGREENS & SPROUTS: These zippy little guys have a ton of flavor and are a fantastic supplement to your Bowl. Look around at your local grocery store and give a few a try. They are both cute and tasty!

COLORFUL VEGGIES: Spiralized carrots and beets are a gorgeous addition to your Beast Bowl. Get fancy and buy a spiralizer. Radishes and tomatoes are some other colorful additions that I always keep in the fridge.

AROMATICS: Cilantro, green onions, parsley… fresh herbs of any kind, really. Aromatics add a flavor punch to any Beast Bowl.

MACRONUTRIENT #1 – LEAN PROTEIN

This is my favorite macronutrient group. Ahh… you too? After a base of colorful, leafy micronutrients, protein is the second most important thing to put into your Beast Bowl. Protein keeps you full, helps control blood sugar, and gives you what you need to build those sexy muscles. But how much protein should you eat?

This subject can get complicated really quickly, but it doesn't have to be hard at all. The key is getting enough protein for you. "Enough" could be anywhere from three to eight ounces per meal. Did you know that eating too much protein in one meal can lead to the same sort of nasty insulin spike that sugar causes?

Eating a small to moderate amount of protein per meal is essential if you want to keep your hormones balanced and keep your weight in a healthy range. If you're trying to lose body fat, aim to eat a moderate amount of protein with each meal. If you need to pack on some muscle, then eating a larger serving of protein helps to drive insulin up and encourages the storage of protein.

I eat about four ounces of chicken, beef, or pork, or six ounces of seafood, in each of my Bowls. This amounts to about one-half to three-quarters of a cup of protein per Bowl. If you are following a plant-based lifestyle, you can substitute firm tofu or tofu crumbles in many of the recipes.

MACRONUTRIENT #2 — HEALTHY FATS

We live in a fat-fearing culture. As a nation, we have reduced the amount of fat we eat, only to get fatter and fatter. We've been told some fats are healthy, but we are still afraid to eat any of it. So what's the deal?

When we have too much body fat, it's usually because we have become insulin resistant. Insulin resistance comes from eating too much insulin-inducing food, like sugar and processed carbs, too often. The good news is that insulin resistance can be reversed by reducing the amount of processed carbohydrates (and, in extreme cases, too much protein) in the diet.

Dietary fat, on the other hand, is crucial for building the hormones that fuel our metabolic processes. That's including the process of muscle growth! Fat has almost no impact on blood insulin and can therefore be the preferential macronutrient if we are wanting to get leaner. In other words, eat fatter, get skinnier.

MY FAVORITE HEALTHY FATS

Avocados and avocado oil

Olive oil

Nuts and seeds

The sauces and dressings in this book

MACRONUTRIENT #3 — CARBOHYDRATES

Ahh, the controversial carbohydrate. Are carbs good or bad? Try not to think of any of the macronutrients as good or bad. We all have different dietary needs and we all respond to macronutrient ratios differently. It's important to find what works for you. Blame genetics.

My husband can indulge in processed sugar and baked goods and has almost zero issues with gaining unwanted weight. He maintains his lean frame despite rarely working out and living on mochas and scones. I, on the other hand, have a tendency to be pretty carb intolerant. I gain unwanted weight easily despite working out almost daily and eating next to no processed foods. I build muscle really quickly, and I store fat really easily. My body would have been well suited for surviving most of human history! Thank you, genetics! I have found that a lower-carb diet works better for my body and helps me in maintaining a healthy weight and performance level.

Notice, though, that I didn't say "low carb" or "ketogenic." When I experimented with extremely low carb diets, I found that my strength suffered drastically. For months, I struggled to back squat 165 pounds. After I upped my carbs from under 50 grams a day to around 200 grams a day, I found I was able to squat 285 pounds less than a month later. Carbs are no joke. More power!!!

Here's the trick to carbohydrates. Eat them in the right amounts at the right times. Also, lift heavy weights. That's it.

Now here's the complicated backstory. Carbohydrates are a quick energy source. They provide the energy that your body needs to fuel intense activities, especially quick and fast movements like sprints or Olympic lifting. Carbohydrates are like turbo boosters for your muscles.

But excess carbohydrates will typically be stored as body fat. When you have a bunch of pesky excess carbohydrates hanging around, you lose the benefit of eating all those carbs in the first place. You want to eat only as many carbs as your muscles need to use, and you want to eat those carbs close to the time that your muscles will be using them, usually within a two-hour window before or after you work out. You don't want those suckers hanging out as sugar in your bloodstream just waiting for some insulin to start up the storage cues.

Our bodies are extremely smart, and they will adapt in order to burn whatever energy source we are eating. If we eat no carbs, our bodies burn fat. If we eat a sufficient or excess amount of carbs, our bodies will burn carbs. While this is generally the case, remember that genetics can also play a role in which one is better for our specific physiological makeup.

This brings us to keto. As of the publishing of this book, the ketogenic diet is the hot fad diet of the moment. In the loosest terms, keto is a high-fat diet that is low in protein and carbs. There can be a time and a place for keto. However, like most diets that call out one or more of the macronutrients as bad, this diet can be hard to maintain long term. Some people are better genetically adapted for a keto diet. Some of us are not. The key is finding what balance of micronutrients works for your body.

Finding that place where your body can just hang out and maintain a healthy weight requires balanced hormones. Hormones are complicated and also not so complicated. Our twenty-first century lifestyle has left most of us with, shall I say, less than ideal hormone profiles. There are so many factors involved here... too much sitting, too much computing, too much food that comes in packages, not enough sun, not enough exercise. And that's not to mention the big stuff like stress, sleep or lack thereof, genetics, and gut health.

All these things affect your insulin levels, not by exactly the same means, but with the same end result — weight gain that is hard as heck to get rid of.

FINDING THE RIGHT BALANCE FOR YOU

The biggest determinant of body composition and leanness is whether or not you are eating the right amount of food for you. So yes, calories do play a role here, but not in the way you may have been told. Cutting calories simply does not work long term for healthy weight management. Sure, you can starve yourself for a few months, but you're not going to maintain that weight loss. It has been proven over and over again. Eating moderate amounts of protein, high-fiber carbs like fruits and vegetables, and healthy fat is more effective than just cutting calories.

The one thing that is crucial for getting leaner is spending more time in a lower insulin state. This can be accomplished in a few ways.

Yes, following a ketogenic diet is one way that you can spend more time in a lower insulin state. Keto allows you to consume a large volume of food that is low in insulin-spiking macronutrients (fat), which can be great for a period of time. However, I'm not sure that this lifestyle is fully sustainable long term. And again, if you're trying to make gains in the gym, you may even find it hard to see desirable progress while adhering to a strict ketogenic diet.

The second way is the practice of fasting, popularly known as "IF," or intermittent fasting. In IF, you basically take a break from feeding yourself for a longer time period than what seems normal in our Western culture. People have really strong opinions about fasting. However, the fact is that fasting has been practiced all over the world for centuries, and there are many health benefits associated with fasting.

Some of these benefits can include the release of those hormones that encourage muscle building. There have also been studies that practitioners of IF have very positive strength gains.

IF protocols can vary from just skipping breakfast to skipping several days of eating. Fasting can be a powerful tool in weight loss, but it should only ever be approached from a healthy mindset. I use IF with my clients when they have a difficult time determining when they are hungry. Fasting can help you lean into that hunger just a little bit.

So what do you do? How do you figure all of this out?

First, you must stop obsessing about every single calorie and macronutrient and find a way to enjoy eating! Relax and nourish yourself.

Rediscovering the joy of eating is what *Beast Bowl Nutrition* is all about. Every Bowl has a balanced amount of all the things that you need to feel satisfied after eating, completely customizable for your individual nutritional needs. You can let go of excessively strict macro counting and build a balanced meal that is good for you and tastes good, too.

It's important to have a general idea about the amounts that you are eating of protein, carbs, and fats. But it's just as necessary to listen to your hunger cues and figure out when you need to eat and when you've eaten enough.

A FEW BASIC GUIDELINES TO KEEP IN MIND:

Don't get super hung up on numbers and macros.

Pay attention to your hunger signals. Eat when you get hungry, and stop eating when you are satisfied. **NOT FULL — BUT SATISFIED.**

Adjust the amount of lean protein and carbs in your Beast Bowl to fit your needs. Believe it or not, once you figure out how to listen to it, your body will tell you what it needs.

When you need some help, head over to FoodologyGeek.com/BBN — I have lots of tips and resources to help keep your meal prep game on point.

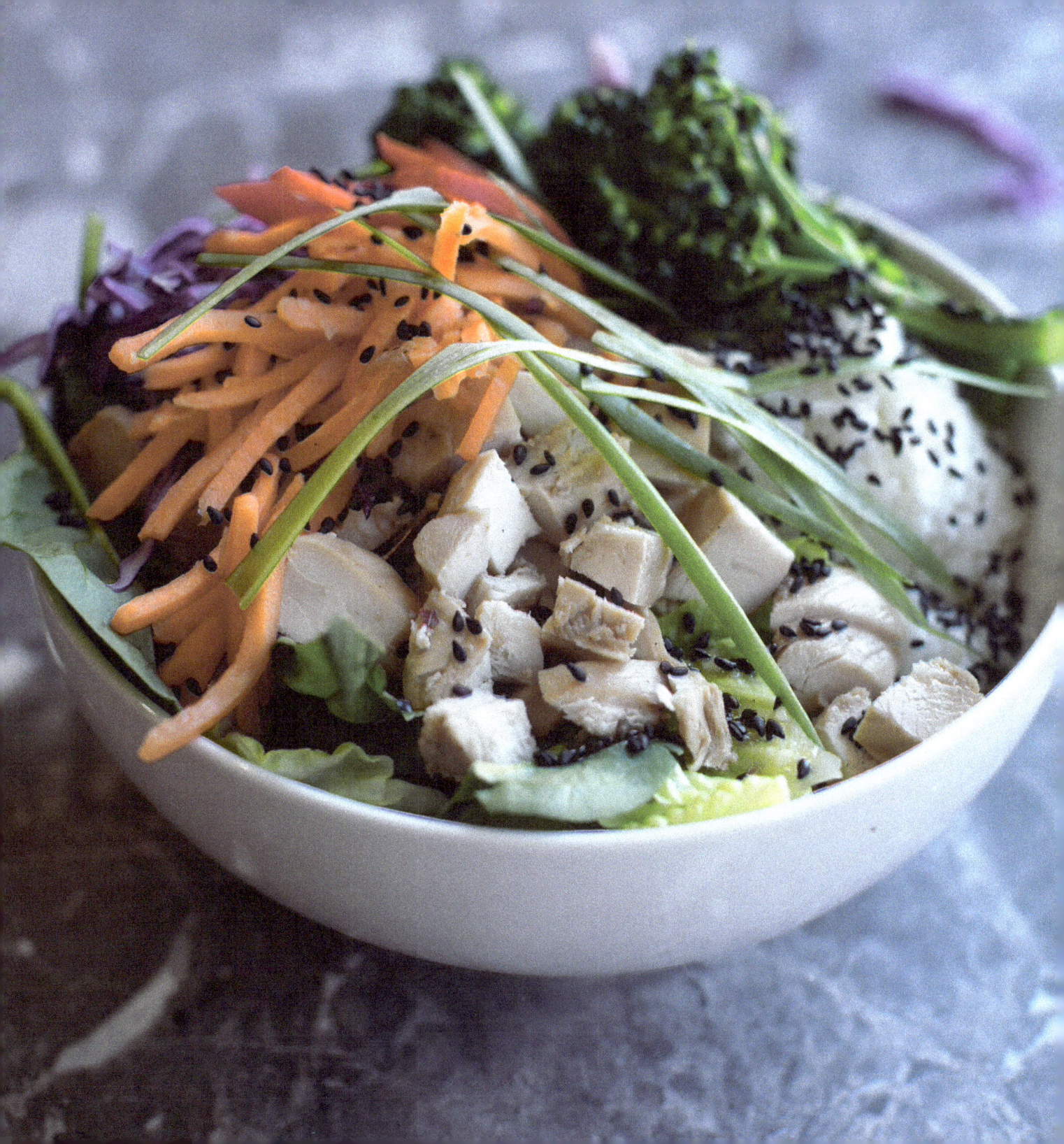

CHAPTER 2
BUILDING A BOWL

One Bowl = Endless Possibilities

What's in your Beast Bowl?

This chapter breaks down the basics of a Beast Bowl in a step-by-step pictorial lesson. For this example, we're going to use the Teriyaki Beast Bowl, but the concepts apply to all the Beast Bowls in this book. Be creative and use the basics to start building a healthy diet one Bowl at a time.

There is no "right" way to build a Beast Bowl. Your Beast Bowl can be anything you want it to be. The only rules are that it should taste fantastic and that you should love eating it.

Beast Bowls are designed to make eating healthfully super easy. If you follow the basic idea of (a few handfuls of colorful veggies) + (the "right" size serving of protein) + (top it off with a healthy serving of fat) + (get some carbs when you need them), building a healthy meal becomes very simple.

Eating this way allows you to get the approximate right amounts and balance of nutrients without spending all day measuring and weighing.

1. THE BOWL

It all starts with a bowl. Find a large bowl that you love. It should be big. You should be able to stuff a bunch of healthy food into it and then toss it around before you shovel everything into your face.

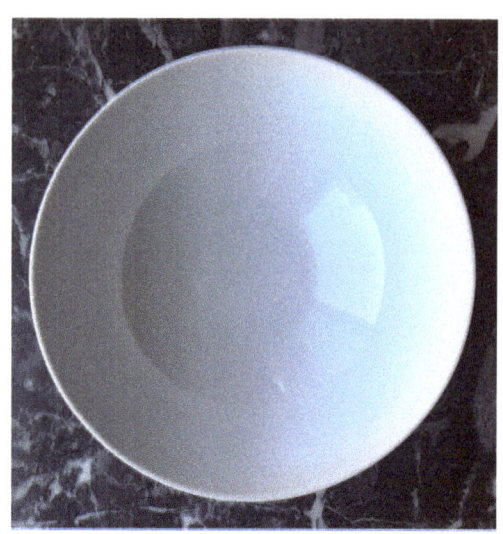

2. ONE HANDFUL OF GREENS

Pick a few different greens to fill up your bowl. A few suggestions are romaine lettuce, baby kale, lacinato kale, spinach, and spring greens.

Throw in anything you like and are willing to chew. If you are having trouble getting in a ton of greens at first, then just start slowly. Eat one big handful and be okay with that. The goal here is to move closer and closer to the best choice. However, don't beat yourself up if you can't do that all at once. Do what you can today! Celebrate a tiny win!

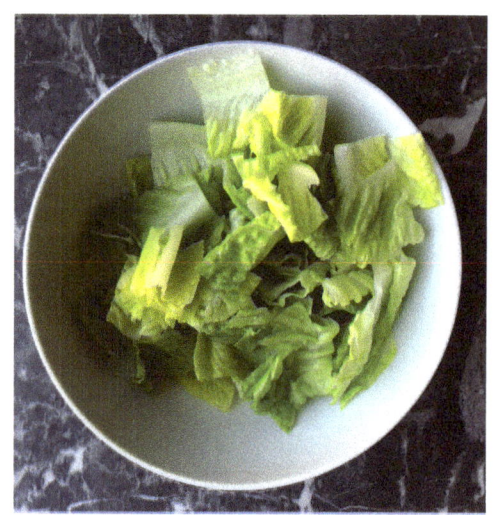

BEAST BOWL NUTRITION | CHAPTER 2 | BUILDING A BOWL

3. THE SECOND HANDFUL OF GREENS – YUM!

The same advice for the first handful applies to the second handful. Here you see two relatively easy-to-eat greens, romaine lettuce and baby spinach.

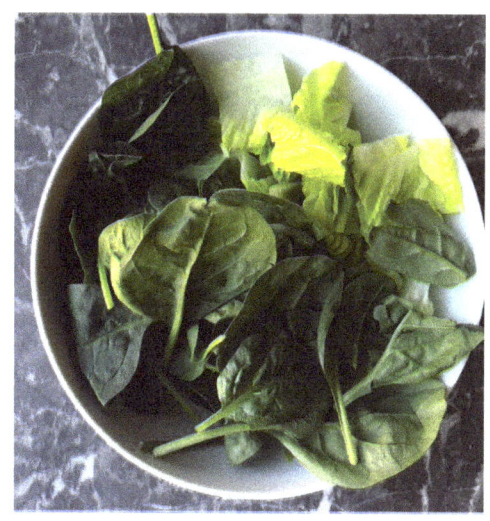

4. DRESSING = SOME HEALTHY FAT

Every Beast Bowl has a delicious sauce or dressing. These sauces and dressings are one of my favorite ways to add some healthy fat to my diet. I usually mix up a batch of dressing that goes with whatever core protein I am eating that week.

Using a small Mason jar makes quick work of mixing up a vinaigrette. A whisk or mini food processor is perfect for making a mayo-based sauce.

Choose healthy fats like coconut oil, nut oil, olive oil, or avocado oil.

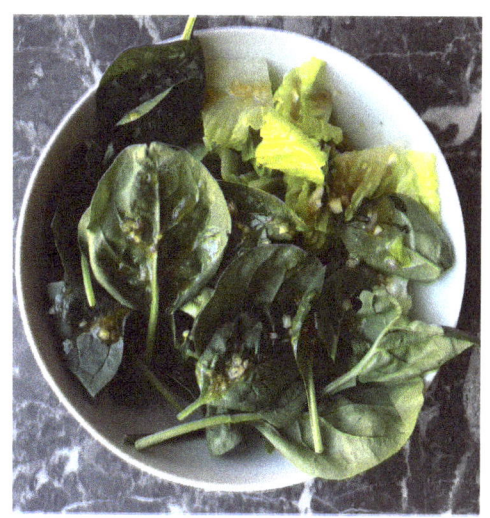

5. A FEW CARBS WHEN YOU NEED THEM

My go-to carbs are white or brown rice, quinoa, and white or sweet potatoes. It's generally best to eat carbs within two hours of when you might work out.

Again, everyone is different. If you find that you are gaining more weight than you would like, you can try adjusting the amount of carbs that you are eating. I recommend giving it about two weeks to notice if this adjustment is helping you.

When my clients are struggling with a plateau, the first thing I have them try is cutting down on carbs. We often have too much blood sugar floating around, and cutting down on carbs for a period of time can help get this problem in check. Then you can start to add carbohydrates back in to your diet at a rate that works for your metabolism and activity level.

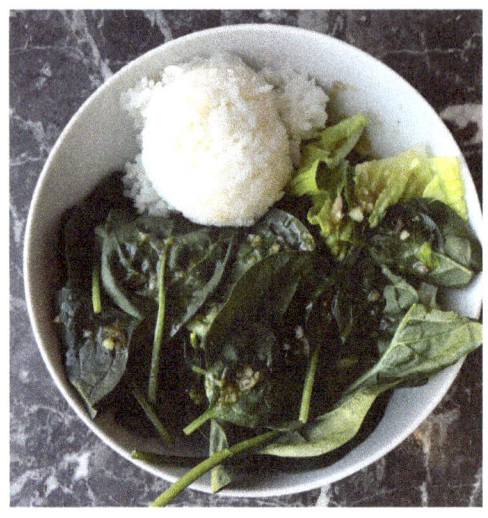

6. GETTING YOUR CORE PROTEIN

The core protein is the heart of the Beast Bowl and the heart of meal prep. Protein is the main building block for lean muscle mass. If you want lean muscle mass, you have to eat protein in the right amounts.

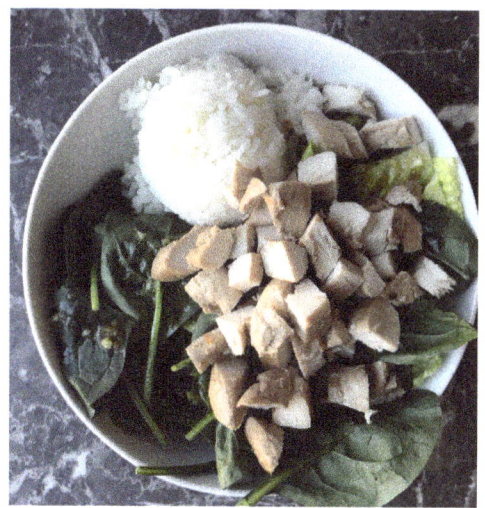

I recommend getting at least three ounces of lean protein at every meal. Larger-framed, athletically-built people may need up to eight ounces of protein per meal. Protein requirements vary depending on your genetics and the type of workouts you are including in your lifestyle. This usually means a quality meat or seafood source. Eggs are also a great source of protein. Vegetarian sources can include tofu and soy products, although I do not recommend eating a diet that is heavy in soy for many reasons.

As mammals, we assimilate animal protein more efficiently than plant protein. This does not mean that plant protein is not a good source of protein. It just means that if you're choosing a plant-based lifestyle, some supplementation might be required to get enough quality protein. There are a lot of supplements to choose from that include plant-based protein. Rice and pea protein are two very common alternatives to whey and other animal proteins.

I have to confess that I encourage my vegetarian clients to include eggs in their diets. Ideally, I like to see them on an ovo-pescatarian diet, which includes fish and eggs. Both of these are solid choices of protein and contain a substantial amount of healthy fats. Win-win!

7. MORE COLOR

I try to add as many different colors to my Beast Bowl as possible. Here is some red cabbage for crunch. Sometimes I just slice up whatever fresh veggies I may have on hand and throw them on top, and other times I pre-prep a flavorful slaw that keeps all week in the fridge.

There are a ton of different slaws and salsas. These pre-prepped options are a great way to add flavor and texture to your Beast Bowl. If you are meal prepping for the week, it helps to spend about twenty minutes cutting up all your veggies and packing them in containers so that you don't have to deal with them for the rest of the week.

Cut once, pack once, clean up once. It really does save time. The first time you meal prep, it might seem overwhelming. But once you have a few weeks of meal prep under your belt, you will have it figured out. Like everything in life, it just takes practice. Get in there and flex your meal prep muscle.

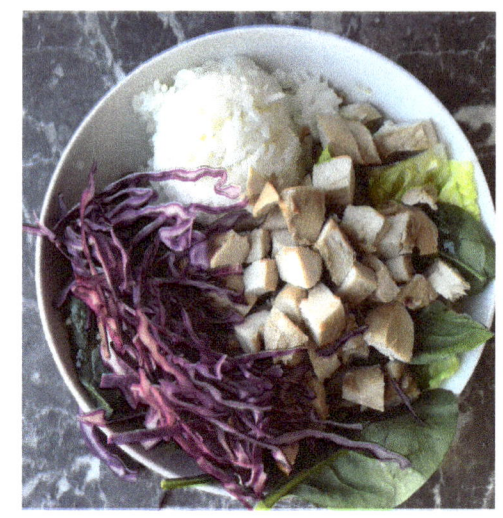

8. AND EVEN MORE COLOR

Ooh...

Crunchy carrots.

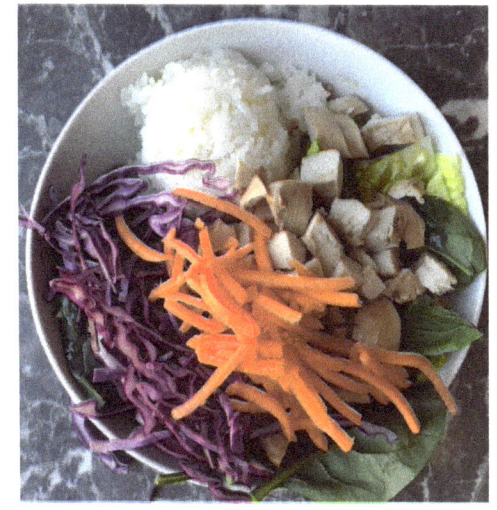

9. AND STILL MORE COLOR

Ahh...

Crisp red bell pepper.

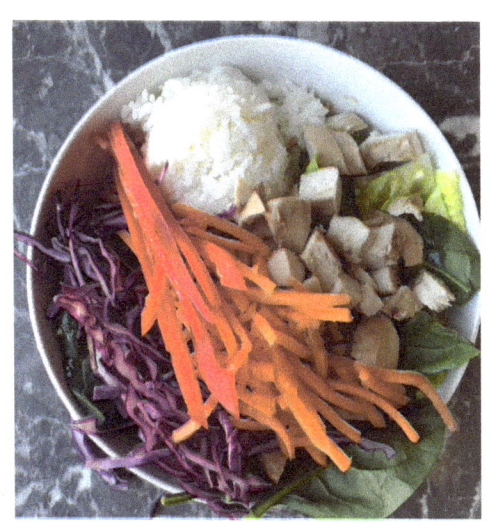

10. BIG FLAVOR

I love to add big flavor to my Beast Bowls in the form of fresh herbs. Green onions, cilantro, and basil are some of my favorites. There is no end to the flavors that you can add here.

Sprouts and microgreens are also great options. Keep an eye out for these guys because they're delicious! These tiny little greens will take your Beast Bowl into the gourmet stratosphere. You so fancy!

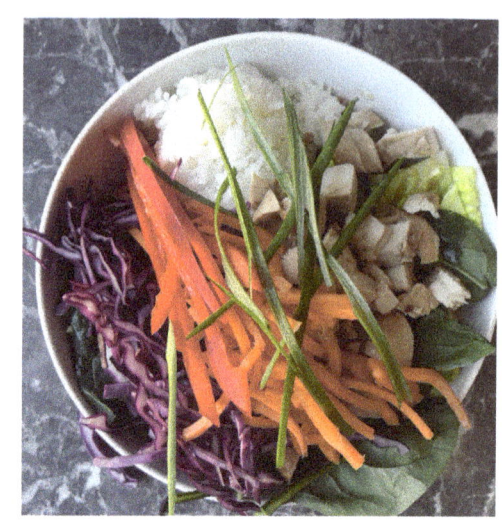

11. ADD THE EXTRAS

A lot of times when I meal prep, I pre-cook the veggies that I will be eating during the week. This can even include broccoli, if you want. Steaming or roasting a batch or two of veggies will ensure that you are prepared and armed with an arsenal of goodies that you can easily throw in your Bowl.

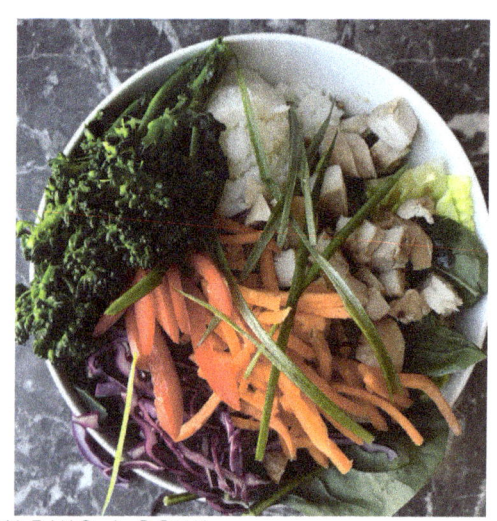

12. FLAVOR 101

Because I'm all about flavor, I try to add a little something extra. Here, I add sesame seeds. I might add some soy sauce or tamari, or maybe even a little extra dressing.

Eating Beast Bowl-style gives me an endlessly flexible way of eating that makes me relatively confident that I am eating what my body needs.

I know that everything that goes into every Bowl is an unprocessed whole food, and I follow the rules of building a badass Beast Bowl when I am hungry. Then I eat it mindfully, savoring every delicious bite, and I stop when I start to feel satisfied.

I guarantee that when you practice eating this way, it will take the stress out of eating for you, too.

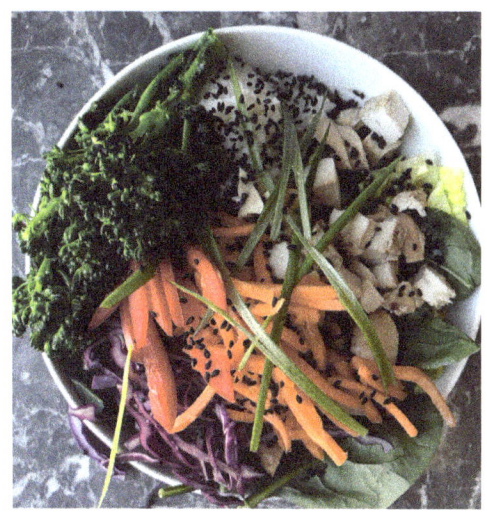

FINALLY: EVERY BOWL IS ADAPTABLE

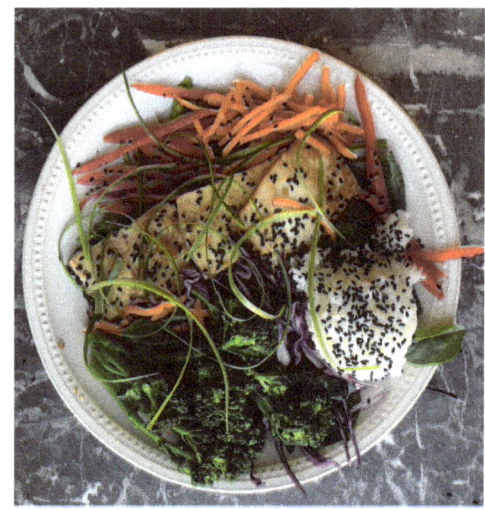

I modified this Bowl for my vegan daughter. It's easy to use the Teriyaki Marinade to sauté up a few slices of extra firm tofu.

I could have used salmon or shrimp here. The Teriyaki Marinade is also great on steak. Keep in mind that every Beast Bowl in the book is just one possible version of the meal. Each marinade is versatile, and you can use it on more than one type of protein. If you like chimichurri but don't eat steak — no problem, chimichurri tastes just as fantastic on shrimp or chicken. Each Bowl recipe includes a suggestion about the type of tweaks that you can make to it.

Remember, almost every recipe is vegan adaptable, but that's not all — these bowls are "protein flexible." Find more ways to mix and match these proteins at FoodologyGeek.com/BBN.

WHAT ABOUT PORTION CONTROL?

Beast Bowl building relies on common sense portion control. What does this mean?

The two most important rules to finding your healthy weight:

1) Only eat when you are hungry.

2) Eat enough food so that you no longer feel hungry.

Okay, that sounds easy. Right? I am sure you know from personal experience that this is a lot harder than it sounds. My clients struggle with this every day. Heck, I struggle with this every day. We are so accustomed to eating on schedule or eating a recommended number of calories that these two rules seem way too fast and loose. But in reality, if you can follow just these two rules, you won't need to do anything else with your diet.

HOW EATING BEAST BOWL-STYLE HELPS WITH PORTION CONTROL

Following the Beast Bowl recipes will automatically give you the correct macronutrient ratios for sensible portions.

So let's review average recommended portions. Keep in mind that these portions are a starting point. If you find that you are gaining more weight or losing more weight than you want, you should adjust the portions to fit your individual lifestyle and metabolism. Everybody is different. There is not a single right way to eat for everyone.

I teach my clients to use visual cues for portions. Why? Because you always have your hands with you. You may not always have a scale or measuring cups and spoons. Plus, it is so much easier.

The reality is that even when you are measuring and weighing every single thing, calorie counting is not an exact science. Our bodies process and use calories differently. A few extra ounces of chicken at one meal does not make or break your body composition.

The real change happens by choosing to eat the right balance of food most of the time and then paying attention to your hunger and satiety cues. Not hungry? Don't eat. Finding yourself starving after a few hours? Add a little more food to each meal.

FOR AN AVERAGE, MODERATELY ACTIVE FEMALE, USE THESE PORTION CONTROL GUIDELINES:

COLORFUL VEGGIES: 2 to 3 large handfuls (about 2 to 3 cups)

PROTEIN: 1 palm-sized portion (about ½ to ¾ cup)

FAT: 1 thumb-sized portion (about 1 tablespoon)

CARBS & FRUIT: 1 cupped handful (about ⅓ cup)

FOR AN AVERAGE, MODERATELY ACTIVE MALE, USE THESE PORTION CONTROL GUIDELINES:

COLORFUL VEGGIES: 4 to 6 large handfuls (about 4 to 6 cups)

PROTEIN: 2 palm-sized portions (about 1 to 1½ cups)

FAT: 2 thumb-sized portions (about 2 tablespoons)

CARBS & FRUIT: 2 cupped handfuls (about ⅔ cup)

WHEN TO MAKE ADJUSTMENTS

If you start feeling hungry less than two hours after you eat, you probably should add a little more food. I recommend adding veggies and protein first. After that, you can add some extra fats. Carbohydrates are best added around workout times. A two-hour window before or after working out is optimal for giving you the right energy when you need it.

If you're NOT feeling hungry after a few hours, you should probably eat a little less food at each meal. I like to adjust down the carbohydrates first, mainly because they are the least micronutrient dense. The colorful veggies and fruits have a lot more bang for their buck when it comes to getting nutrition that counts.

Rice and quinoa may give you energy, but they are a lot less necessary when it comes to keeping your metabolism and hormones running efficiently. Eat these denser carbs with moderation in mind.

The real change happens by choosing to eat the right balance of food most of the time and then paying attention to your hunger and satiety cues. Not hungry? Don't eat. Find yourself starving after a few hours? Add a little more food to each meal.

CHAPTER 3
MEAL PREP 101

Let's Talk Meal Prep

While meal prep does involve a little planning and some practice, it doesn't have to be complicated. The secret to meal prepping with Beast Bowls is to think of each Bowl in terms of its component parts and then to imagine all the ways that you can mix and match those individual parts.

If you hate cooking, focus on making things as simple as possible. Start by picking out one of the protein recipes. Then just make that protein.

All the fixins that go into the Bowl can easily be found pre-packaged, pre-washed, and pre-cut. You can always buy your favorite sides and dressings instead of making them from scratch. Once you get in the habit of prepping your proteins each week, then try making one yummy plant-based extra at home. Baby steps! Get good at one and then add another.

Getting efficient at anything takes practice, and meal prep is no exception. If this is your first time meal prepping, start small. Make one Beast Bowl this week. Once you get really good at that Bowl, then add another.

I APPROACH MY WEEK IN A 1-2-3 SORT OF WAY.

1

I usually make one batch of soup for the week. I know this is a book about Beast Bowls, but I think soup deserves a shout-out in meal prep. Soup is cool! It can hang out with Beast Bowls and fit right in. Having a batch of soup around is an easy way to fill in the gaps when you need extra veggies, or just a snack to hold you over. If you need a few easy soup and stew ideas, check out the lineup of recipes on the blog at FoodologyGeek.com

Often, I simply make a big batch of bone broth. I will sip on a hot cup of broth when I'm hungry and need just a little something warm. Bone broth contains minerals and gut-healing collagen. If you aren't sipping on this stuff, you're missing out on some awesome health benefits.

The leftover chicken from the bone broth can be shredded and eaten on top of a slaw or a bed of veggies. You can also whip up a quick mayo and add your favorite seasoning mix to make it into a chicken salad.

2

Next, I pick two proteins. I start by picking two Beast Bowl recipes that I want to make, then I know which proteins I will be making for the week. Sometimes I just make the proteins from the Beast Bowl recipe and then eat that protein right out of the fridge with an apple and a few almonds. I know it's not fancy, but I'm busy and I've got to eat.

When planning your meals for the week, you can easily figure out how much of each core protein you will need to prep. You just need to decide how many servings you want to make of each protein, and how many ounces you need for each serving. Multiply them together and you have your total ounces to prep.

$$\text{number of servings for the week} \times \text{ounces of protein per serving} = \text{number of ounces to prep}$$

EASY, RIGHT?

When planning out my prep for the week, I start by picking two different Beast Bowls from the lineup, each with a different core protein. I plan to make two meals with each core protein, plus enough for leftovers. As an example, here's the math for a family of 4. 8 servings + 4 servings of leftovers, for a total of 12 servings per protein. Each person in the family might eat 4 to 6 ounces of protein with each meal. So if I'm planning for Asian Chicken Meatballs, I need to prep 4 x 12 = 48 ounces (3 pounds) of chicken.

For two Beast Bowl recipes and a family of four, you would need to prep six to eight pounds of protein each week.

3

My last step is to select the three vegetable options that I'll use throughout the week. This is where the extras in the Beast Bowls come in. Typically, if you pick two Beast Bowl recipes for the week and make the suggested extras, you should end up with enough veggies to get in all ten of your servings each day. A lot of the extras in this book are slaws and salsas. Each one gives your Beast Bowl not only a massive hit of fresh, crunchy flavor and texture but also gives you a good-sized portion of veggies and/or fruits.

Remember, focus at first on just making the protein in each Bowl. The rest of the extras and dressings are the bling. Add them to your meal prep rotation when you feel competent with making the proteins each week. Until then, don't sweat it... do the best you can and enjoy the delicious proteins with some veggies on the side.

MEAL PREP DAY INCLUDES:

Start by planning out your week. Decide what veggies you'll need to chop to use for cooking right now and what veggies you will pack into containers to use later in the week.

Cook any proteins that you have planned for the week. Make sure to bring meat to room temp before you start cooking, so that your cooking times are accurate.

Make any extras and/or sauces.

Remember, taking shortcuts is totally fine. I like to make all of my sauces and extras from scratch. But I'm kinda weird like that. I love cooking, what can I say?

If you don't like cooking as much as I do, then you'll need to strategize. What things can you buy pre-made? It doesn't have to be perfect. Being healthy is all about having an approach that is sustainable for you! That starts with making the best possible choice for you given your current circumstances.

PRO TIP: Make sure you download the meal planning prep sheet from the blog. It will help you pull all the details together. Find it at FoodologyGeek.com/BBN

The beauty of Beast Bowls is that they are all built with swappable extras and fixins that can be mixed and matched. Each Beast Bowl is created with customization in mind. The published recipe is my version. I give the recipes to you the way I would typically pair and eat them, but you can make them any way you like.

WE ALL NEED SHORTCUTS

Frozen meats are my saving grace. I use a lot of frozen chicken tenderloins and frozen pre-portioned fish when I'm meal prepping. Grass-fed ground beef and ground chicken or turkey are also great to keep in the freezer.

PRO TIP: I buy three to four pounds of meat at a time. This ensures that I have enough protein for the whole week. You can also have your butcher split the meat into two packages. Then you can freeze one for later in the week or save it for another week.

THAWING: To thaw meat extra quickly, place it in a zip-top freezer bag. Place the whole thing in a large bowl of warm water. This method will shorten the time it takes the meat to thaw.

Otherwise, set the meat in the fridge the night before to thaw overnight.

MY FIVE ALWAYS-MUST-HAVE PROTEINS:

Chicken tenderloins (buy them frozen, they thaw quickly)

Grass-fed ground beef (or ground chicken or turkey)

Hanger steaks

Seafood (salmon, halibut or cod, shrimp)

Roasts (pork shoulder or beef chuck)

EXTRAS SHORTCUTS

With practice, you'll get faster at making your own extras. But even if you don't have a ton of time, you can still eat healthfully. It just requires some planning. Remember to go easy on yourself. Do the best you can right now!

If you hate prep work, don't kill yourself over it. Make things easy and plan to buy pre-cut vegetables. This can save a good hour on prep day. All the cleaning, peeling, and scrubbing (not to mention the cleanup!) takes time. Sure, pre-prepped veggies are a little more expensive, but time is money. If you have the money, save the time.

Shredded cabbage and carrots are easy to find. Shredded broccoli can go into any slaw.

Pre-diced veggies and fruits are readily available in the produce section. Pre-made salsa and guacamole are usually in the same section.

Pre-diced butternut squash and sweet potatoes are generally easy to find. Many stores even have mixes of pre-prepped vegetables that are great for roasting or stir-frying and then adding to your Beast Bowl.

The other great thing about the slaws and salsas in this book is that they keep really well in the fridge. Sometimes a pre-done salad will get all wilted in a few days. Not these recipes. They stay nice and crunchy, and their flavor gets even better with time.

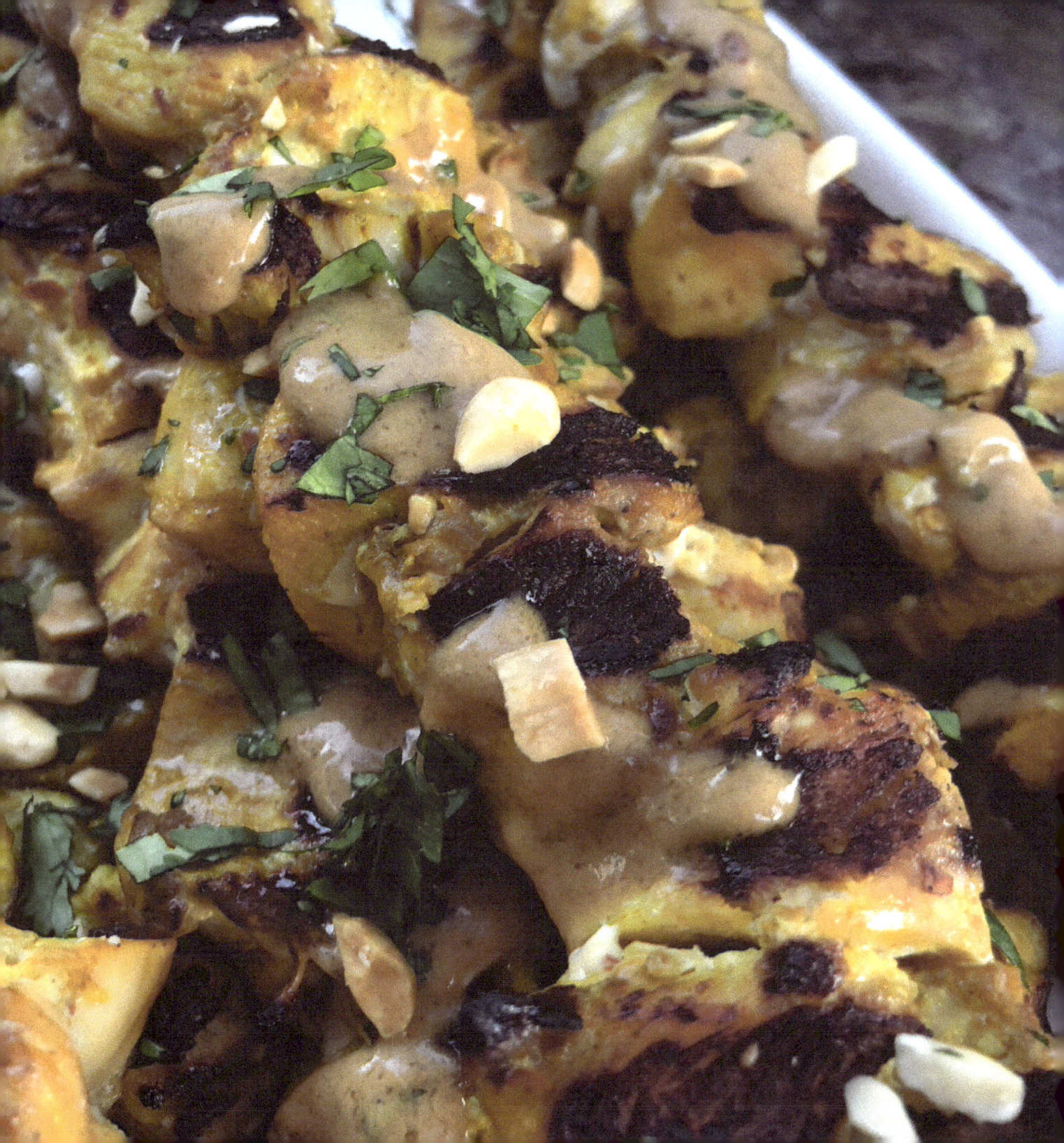

CHAPTER 4
CORE PROTEINS & EXTRAS

The Beast Bowls

Before we dive into the Beast Bowls, let me just say a few things.

I want you to think about each Beast Bowl in terms of its main protein. The Beast Bowl concept of meal prep is meant to be flexible. If you're a beginner, make it easy on yourself and just focus on prepping proteins. Add in extras and dressings as you get better at meal planning and more comfortable with cooking.

The Beast Bowl recipes are meant to get you started thinking about possibilities. The components in each bowl are built to be mixed and matched. Each Beast Bowl in this chapter contains a core protein recipe that serves as the foundation of each bowl. The core proteins are paired with suggested extras and a dressing or sauce. These serving suggestions are just that — suggestions.

These recipes are designed to be super easy and flexible. Many of the marinades and seasoning mixes are delicious on more than one type of protein. For example, the Teriyaki Marinade could be used on chicken, beef, or even with salmon and tofu. Make the Beast Bowls as they were designed and then, once you have a few favorites, try switching up the protein. There is endless flexibility built into these recipes.

All right, let's get started!

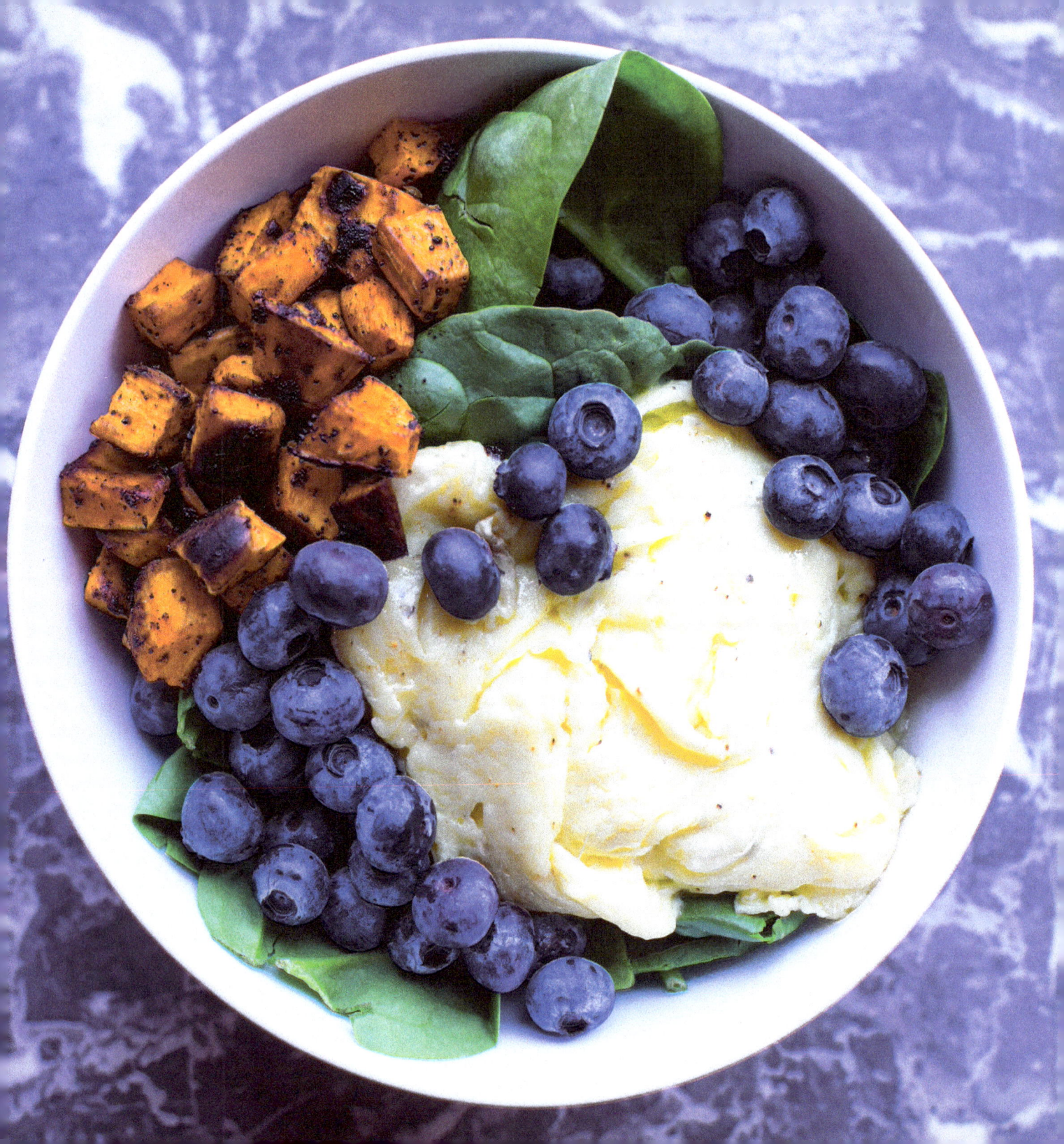

PALEO BREAKFAST

MAKES 1 SERVING

Breakfast can be one of the most challenging meals of the day. Whether you're rushing to get kids to school or yourself to work, who has time to cook in the morning? This super filling breakfast Beast Bowl provides all the protein that you need and a colorful helping of fruits and veggies.

Sweet potatoes are one of my mainstay carb sources, so I usually have a batch in the fridge. They can be pre-roasted so you can just toss them in when you're ready to eat. Another time-saving tip is to make up a batch of baked eggs in muffin cups. In the morning you can reheat them in the microwave for 30 seconds, add your other ingredients, and you've got breakfast!

INGREDIENTS

- 1 to 2 teaspoons butter or avocado oil
- 3 eggs
- ¼ cup egg whites or 1 additional whole egg
- ½ teaspoon Kosher salt
- ¼ teaspoon black pepper

FIXINS

- ½ cup blueberries
- 1½ cup spinach
- ½ cup roasted sweet potatoes /131 (Leftovers are great here.)
- Crispy bacon, made ahead

DIRECTIONS

Heat a skillet on medium. Add 1 to 2 teaspoons butter or oil.

Add the eggs, salt, and pepper to a bowl and whisk.

Cook the eggs in the skillet.

Use a flat spatula to move the eggs around to get a nice scramble.

I add some extra egg whites for some additional protein. This is totally optional.

NOTES

PREP FOR THE WEEK: Use 12 eggs and 1 cup of egg whites. Chop your spinach and mix it right into your eggs with the salt and pepper. Use a muffin pan (a silicone one works well for this). Bake at 350°F for about 20 minutes. Oven temperatures may vary, so make sure you check in on them.

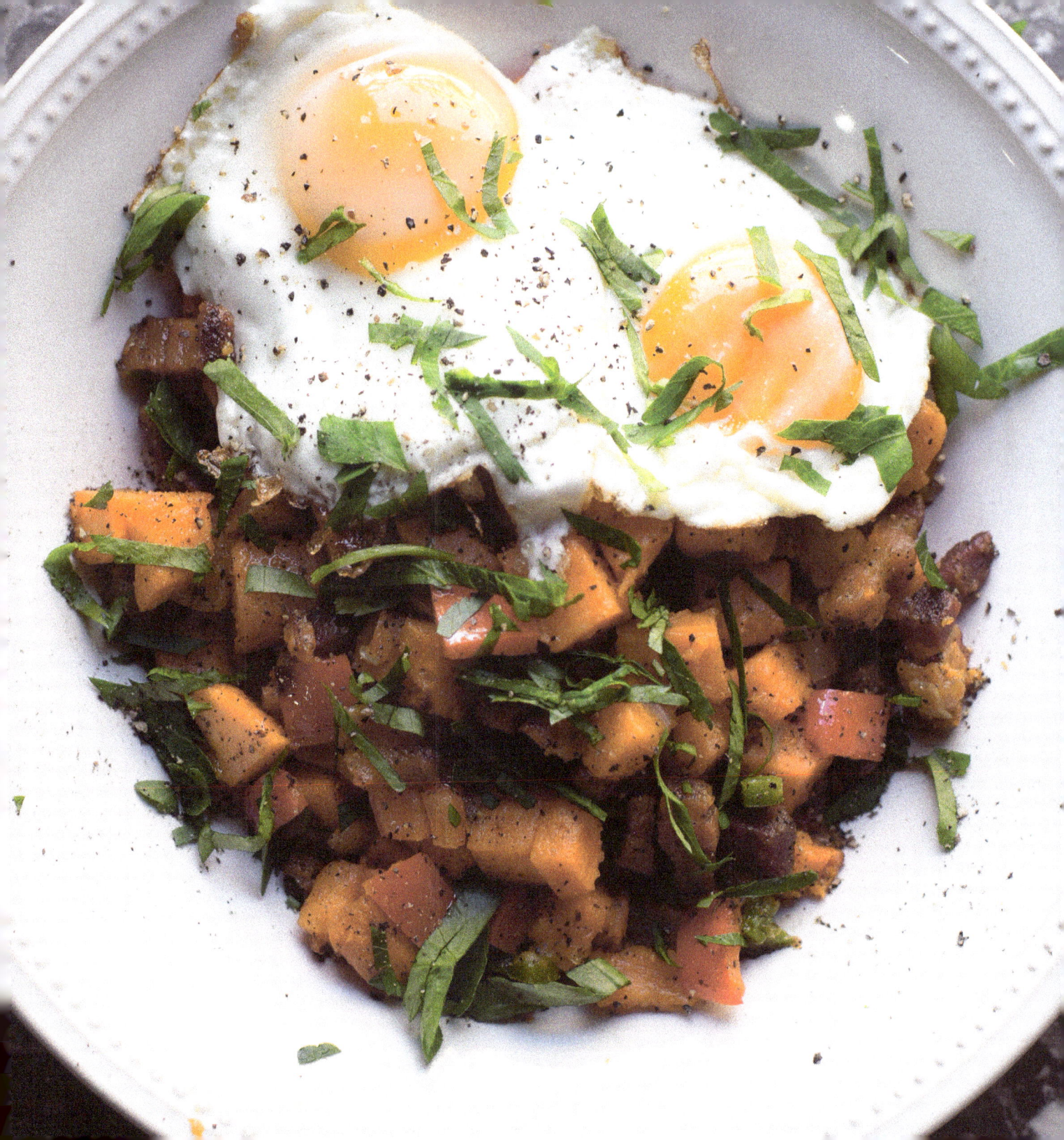

BREAKFAST HASH

MAKES 6 TO 8 SERVINGS

Hash is a beautiful thing. Is there any better way to start off your morning than with crispy, flavorful potatoes just chillin' with salty pancetta? This is a sweet potato hash, but you could also make it with Yukon Gold potatoes. Top it off with a few perfectly cooked eggs, and it's morning plate heaven.

Just bring me a cuppa joe and a good book, and I can make this morning last until afternoon.

INGREDIENTS

- 1 pound pancetta, diced
- 2 pounds sweet potatoes, diced
- 1 yellow onion, diced
- 1 red pepper, diced
- 6 to 12 eggs
- 2 tablespoons fresh parsley, chopped
- ½ teaspoon Kosher salt
- ¼ teaspoon black pepper

DIRECTIONS

Dice the pancetta and brown it over medium heat in a heavy-bottomed skillet.

Remove the pancetta and set it aside. Reserve the grease.

Add the diced sweet potatoes to the reserved grease and brown them.

Add a little black pepper.

Add the onion and red pepper to the pan and cook until soft.

Adjust the seasoning with salt and pepper.

Reduce the heat to low.

Use a large spoon to create 6 spaces in the potatoes for the eggs. Try to space them out evenly.

Crack 1 egg into each of the spaces.

Cover the pan and cook on low until the eggs are just set.

NOTES

MAKE-AHEAD: Cook the eggs separately. Hard- or medium-boiled eggs are easy to pre-prep and then just toss in your bag when you know you need them. Cooked eggs in the shell do not need to be refrigerated, so they're really easy to pack.

PRO TIP: Buy a thick slice of pancetta at the deli counter. The saltiness of pancetta varies from brand to brand. Taste before salting.

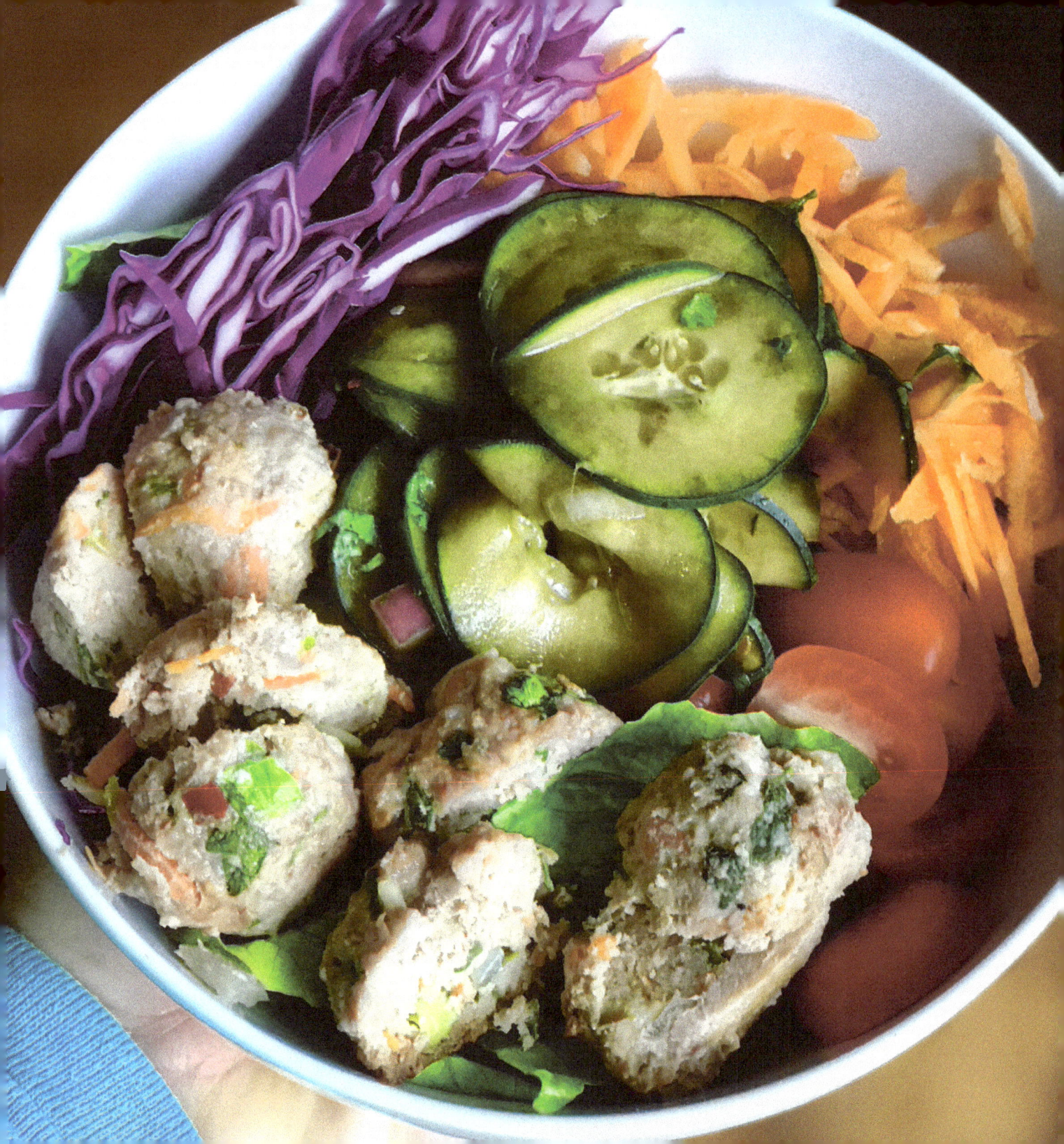

ASIAN CHICKEN MEATBALL

MAKES 6 TO 8 SERVINGS

Meet the very first Beast Bowl! This is even the original photo that went up on Instagram after I made this Bowl. This is typical of how I eat. That particular week, I had made my delicious Asian Chicken Meatballs and some Asian Cucumber Salad. I piled a bunch of veggies into a bowl and then tossed my meatballs and cucumber salad right on top. I finished it with a few tablespoons of Vietnamese Vinaigrette. When I stepped back to look at this magnificent creation, I was like, "That looks like one beast of a bowl!" And the Beast Bowl was born… just like that!

INGREDIENTS

- 2 to 3 pounds ground chicken, turkey, or pork
- ¼ bunch green onions, chopped
- ½ bunch cilantro, chopped
- ¾ cup carrots, shredded
- ¼ red onion, finely diced
- 3 cloves garlic, minced
- 4 teaspoons fresh ginger, minced
- 2 teaspoons chili paste
- 2 tablespoons soy sauce or tamari
- 1½ tablespoons fish sauce, like Red Boat brand
- 1 teaspoon crushed red pepper
- ¼ cup finely ground coconut or almond flour
- 2 eggs

FIXINS

Lettuce
Spinach
Shredded carrots
Green onions
Cilantro

EXTRAS

Asian Cucumber Salad /49
Vietnamese Viniagrette /140

DIRECTIONS

Preheat the oven to 400°F.

Add all the ingredients in a large bowl. Mix well with your hands.

Make the meatballs using your hands or a 2-tablespoon scoop.

Place them on a baking sheet or in a roasting pan.

Bake for 20 minutes total, turning them after about 10 minutes.

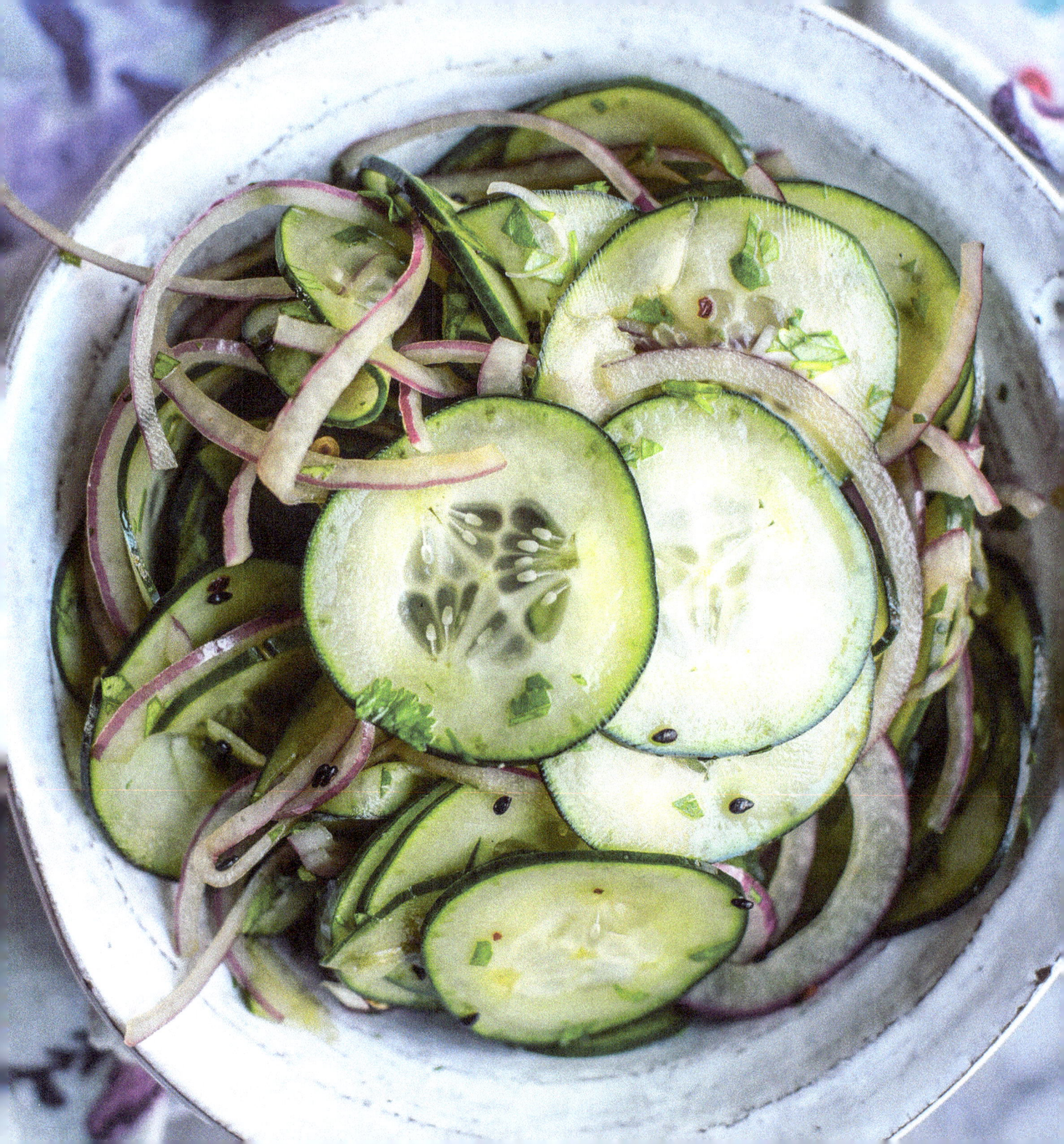

ASIAN CUCUMBER SALAD

INGREDIENTS

3 cucumbers, thinly sliced
½ red onion, thinly sliced

ASIAN DRESSING

¼ cup soy sauce or tamari
¼ cup rice wine vinegar
1 tablespoon mirin
2 teaspoons coconut oil or olive oil
1 clove garlic, pressed
1 teaspoon fresh ginger, grated
1 teaspoon crushed red pepper
¼ bunch cilantro, finely chopped
2 tablespoons sesame seeds (black or white)

DIRECTIONS

Thinly slice the cucumbers and onions.

Add the cucumbers and onions to a large nonreactive bowl.

Combine all of the remaining ingredients to make the dressing.

Pour the dressing over the cucumbers and onions.

Toss to combine.

Store any leftovers in an airtight container in the refrigerator.

For the best flavor, let the salad chill for a few hours before serving.

NOTES

PRO TIP: A mandoline slicer or food processor makes quick work of this.

The Asian Dressing is also great as a quick Asian-style dressing for any lettuce salad.

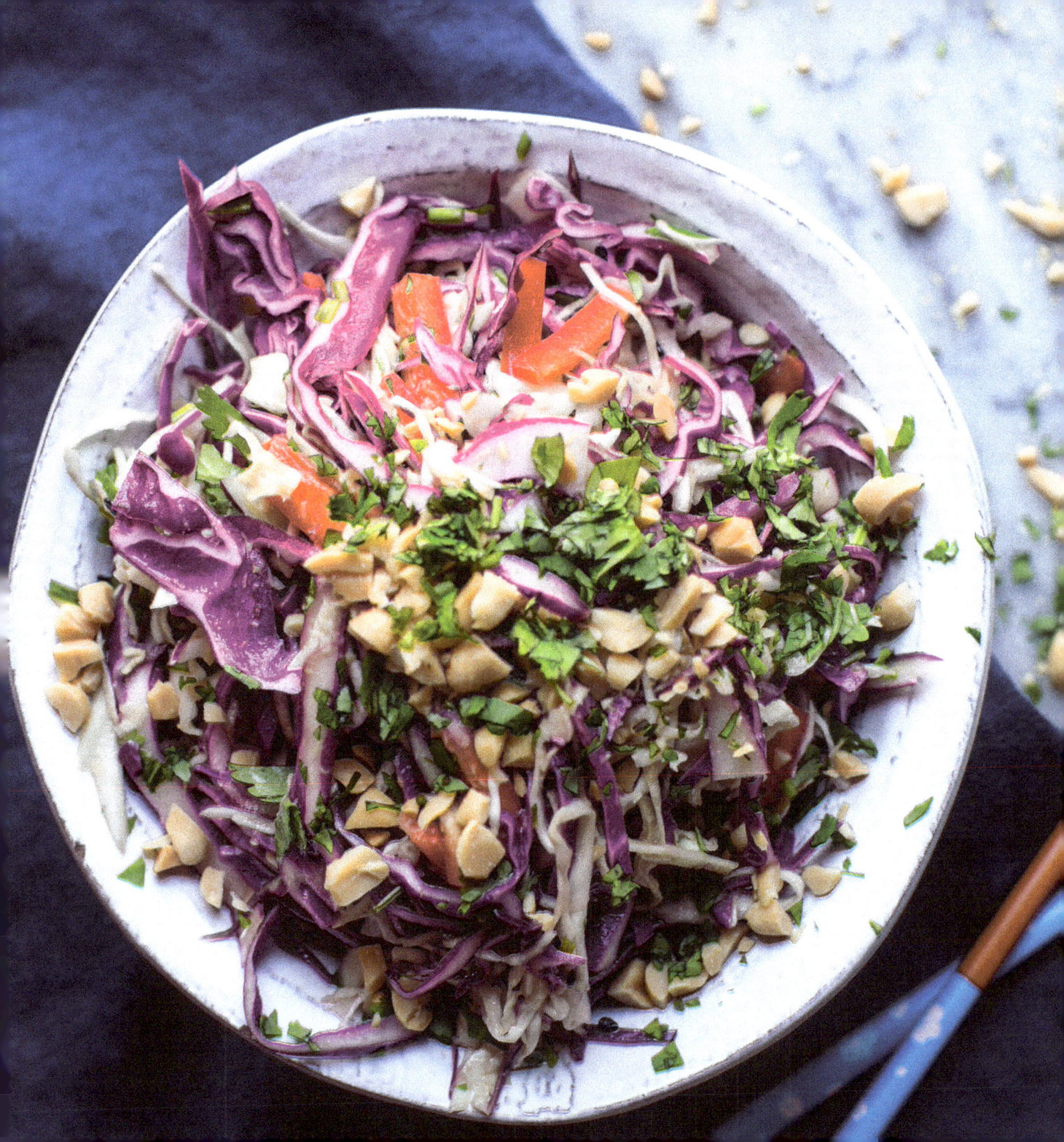

ASIAN SLAW

INGREDIENTS

½ head red cabbage, finely shredded

½ head green cabbage, finely shredded

2 carrots, shredded

1 red bell pepper, finely sliced

½ bunch cilantro, finely minced

1 bunch green onions, thinly sliced

¼ cup roasted peanuts, roughly chopped

ASIAN PEANUT SLAW DRESSING

3 limes, juiced

3 tablespoons creamy, all-natural peanut butter

2 teaspoons fresh ginger, grated

2 tablespoons seasoned rice wine vinegar

2 teaspoons soy sauce

1 to 2 teaspoons fish sauce, like Red Boat brand

1 teaspoon sesame oil

1 tablespoon coconut oil

1 pinch crushed red pepper

1 teaspoon Kosher salt

¼ teaspoon Black pepper

DIRECTIONS

Peel the carrots and shred them. Slice the red bell pepper into thin strips. Slice the cabbage.

In a large bowl, whisk together the lime juice, peanut butter, ginger, rice wine vinegar, soy sauce, fish sauce, sesame oil, and coconut oil. Add in crushed red pepper, salt, and black pepper.

Add the prepared cabbage, carrots, cilantro, green onions, and peanuts to the large bowl with the dressing.

Toss well.

Garnish with chopped peanuts and cilantro.

NOTES

PRO TIP: Use a spiralizer to make noodles out of the carrots and bell pepper.

The Asian Peanut Slaw Dressing is also amazing on any salad, especially with grilled chicken.

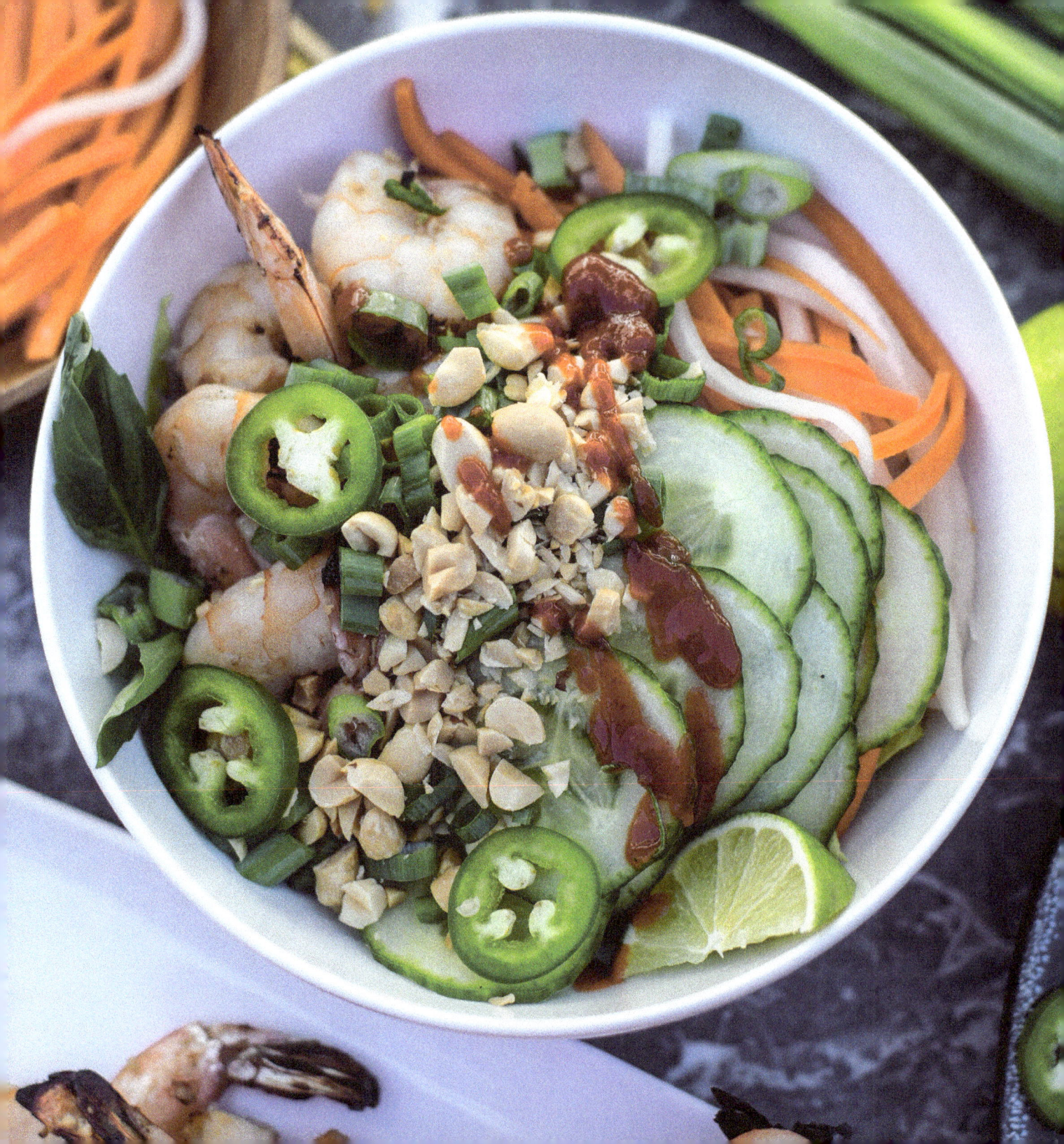

LEMONGRASS SHRIMP

MAKES 6 TO 8 SERVINGS

Vermicelli noodle bowls at my favorite Vietnamese restaurant are one of my favorite meals, but they are usually a little skimpy on the protein and heavier on the rice noodles than I like. While sometimes this is fine, I try to keep things a little lower on the carb side, so I like to make my own version.

This Beast Bowl is full of protein-packed shrimp and served with a ton of fresh vegetables and rice noodles. Pickled carrots and radishes plus Vietnamese Dressing give this Bowl a truly authentic flavor. Don't forget the Sriracha!

INGREDIENTS

2 to 3 pounds shrimp, preferably wild, peeled and deveined

LEMONGRASS MARINADE

2 tablespoons fish sauce, like Red Boat brand
1 teaspoon light brown sugar
3 cloves garlic, minced
1 tablespoon fresh ginger, minced or grated
3 tablespoons finely chopped lemongrass (pale, tender center part only)

FIXINS

Sriracha
Rice noodles, preferably rice vermicelli
Cucumbers, sliced
Roasted peanuts, crushed
Bean sprouts
Lime for squeezing
Lettuce, shredded
Spinach
Mixed herbs: green onions, cilantro, mint, basil

EXTRAS

Asian Cucumber Salad /49
Pickled Asian Veggies /55
Asian Dressing /49

DIRECTIONS

Put the shrimp in a shallow dish.

Add the fish sauce, brown sugar, garlic, ginger, and lemongrass.

Mix well to coat.

Marinate for at least 20 minutes while you are prepping everything else.

If you're making noodles, make them now. Follow the directions on the package.

Shrimp can be sautéed in a pan or grilled.

NOTES

SAUTÉ: Add 1 to 2 tablespoons of oil to a medium-sized pan. Heat to medium-high heat. Add shrimp and cook for 3-5 minutes. The shrimp cook very quickly. They are done as soon as they're pink.

GRILLING: If you're going to grill, place the shrimp on skewers. Don't forget to soak the skewers in water before you use them. Heat your grill to a medium-high flame. Place the skewers on the grill and cook for approximately 2 minutes on each side.

VEGAN ADAPTABLE: Use extra-firm tofu instead of shrimp. Replace the fish sauce with coconut aminos in the dressing and the marinade.

ALTERNATIVE: Substitute chicken or thinly sliced pork tenderloin.

MAKE-AHEAD TIP: The marinade can be prepared ahead of time. Add your protein of choice and store in the refrigerator for a few days or in the freezer for a few weeks.

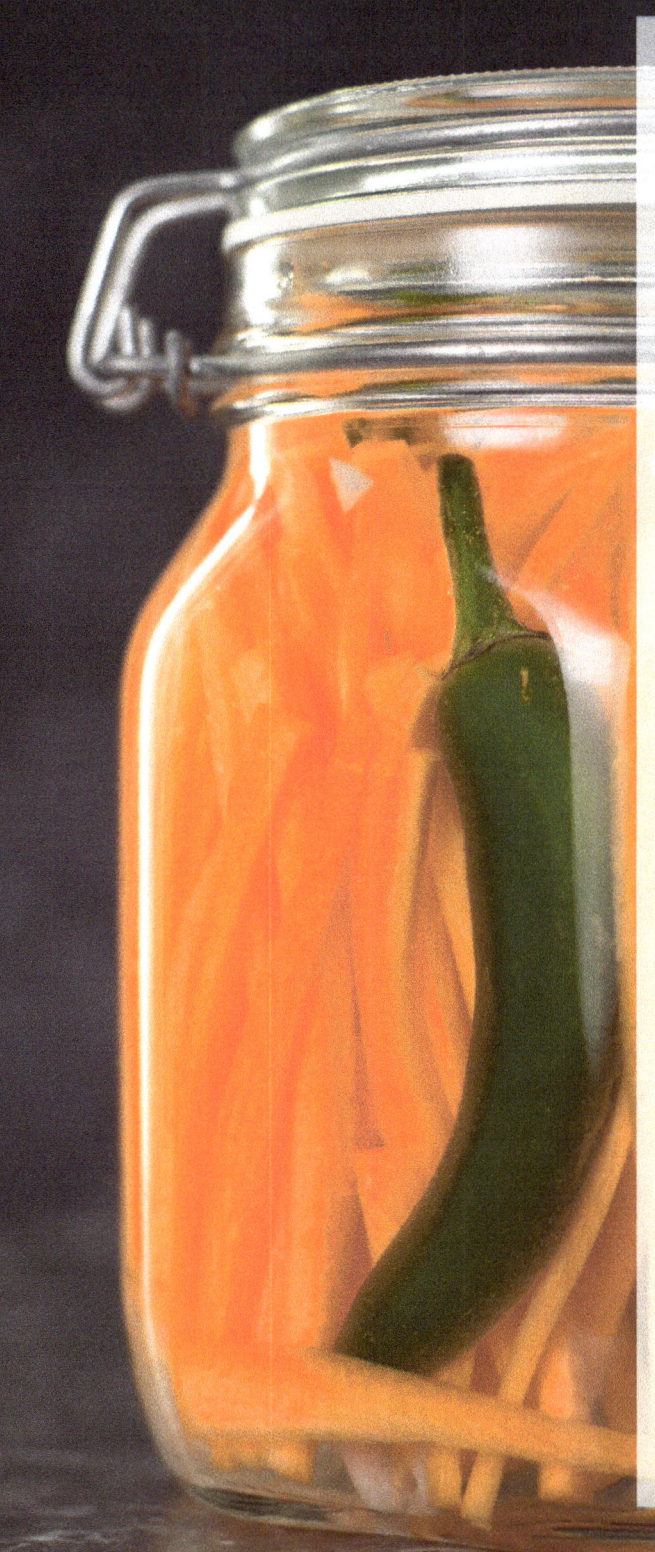

PICKLED ASIAN VEGGIES

INGREDIENTS

1 cup carrots, finely julienned
1 cup daikon, finely julienned
1 to 2 green onions, sliced
1 serrano pepper, sliced in half
2 teaspoons granulated sugar
½ teaspoon Kosher salt
2 tablespoons rice wine vinegar

DIRECTIONS

Peel and cut the carrots and daikon.

Slice the green onions.

Cut the serrano pepper in half.

Combine the sugar, salt, and vinegar in a small bowl. Add to the veggies and toss.

Let sit for about 20 minutes before serving.

To store, place in an airtight container and top off with water to cover.

NOTES

These veggies will keep for a few months in the refrigerator. The flavor keeps getting better in cold storage.

PRO TIP: For best results, use a mandoline slicer fitted with the medium julienne blade.

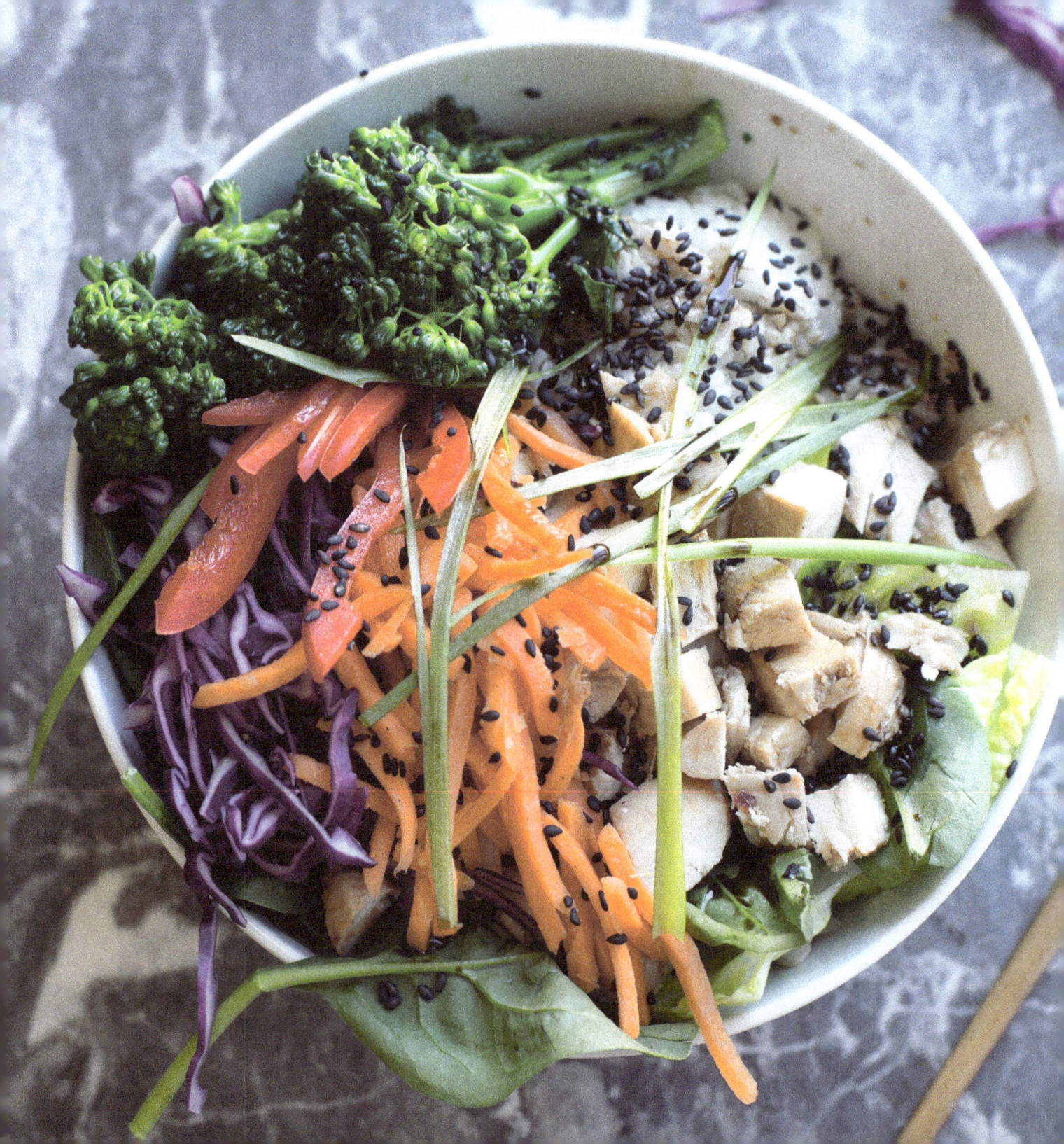

TERIYAKI CHICKEN

MAKES 6 TO 8 SERVINGS

Of all the Beast Bowls here, this one might be the one that I make the most. The Teriyaki Marinade is really easy to make, so I always make a double batch of this stuff. The chicken can be grilled or simply baked in the oven. Crunchy vegetables and rice are a perfect combination! This makes it easy to get all your healthy carbs in. Top it off with sesame seeds and furikake to give this Bowl some nice crunchy bling. The Sesame Ginger Vinaigrette is just a flavor WOW!

INGREDIENTS

2 pounds chicken, breasts or thighs

TERIYAKI MARINADE

2 cloves garlic, minced
2 teaspoons fresh ginger, minced
4 tablespoons soy sauce or tamari
2 tablespoons mirin
2 tablespoons seasoned rice wine vinegar
½ teaspoon crushed red pepper
2 teaspoons brown sugar or honey
1 cup water

FIXINS

White or brown rice
Romaine lettuce
Spinach
Broccoli, blanched
Red pepper, thinly sliced
Red cabbage, thinly sliced
Cucumber, julienned
Carrots, julienned
Green onions, thinly sliced
Sesame seeds
Kimchi
Furikake

EXTRAS

Asian Slaw /51
Asian Cucumbers Salad /49
Sesame Ginger Vinaigrette /147

DIRECTIONS

Add all the ingredients to a gallon-sized freezer bag or a large nonreactive bowl.

Cover or seal and marinate for at least a few hours, up to overnight.

Bake at 425°F for 15 to 20 minutes.

NOTES

ALTERNATIVES: Steak, salmon, or shrimp are delicious in this Bowl.

VEGAN ADAPTABLE: Use extra-firm tofu or portobello mushrooms in place of the chicken.

KIMCHI is full of healthy probiotics that are a must for gut health. I truly love it. Try a few because the flavors can vary widely.

FURIKAKE is a flavorful sprinkle that you add to rice or noodles. You can find it in the Asian section or at Asian grocery stores. If you haven't tried it, you definitely should.

PRO TIP: Marinate the meat overnight in the refrigerator OR marinate it for a few hours at room temperature. A 9x13-inch glass cake pan works really well for this.

GRILL: For steak, grill for about 3 minutes on high heat. For chicken and shrimp, grill for about 6 minutes on medium-high heat.

BROIL: If you're using salmon or another type of fish, broiling is also an option. Place on a broiler pan and broil for 5-7 minutes.

Keep in mind that oven and grill temperatures vary, so make sure you check the timing for your equipment.

HOW TO MEAL PREP IN 5 MINUTES

Meal prep doesn't have to be hard or time-consuming! There are two secrets to effortless meal prep. Number one: Seasoning Mixes because no one wants to eat boring food. Number two: pre-prepped veggies. You can either buy these at your local grocery store or you can spend 30 minutes doing the prep work yourself.

STEP 1: PICK YOUR PROTEIN

Chicken Breasts
Chicken Thighs
Ground Chicken
Hanger Steak
Ground Beef
Salmon
Halibut
Firm Tofu

PRO TIP: Bring all meat to room temp before cooking!

STEP 2: FIND A SEASONING MIX

Barbecue Rub /187
Buffalo Seasoning /186
Herbes de Provence Seasoning /185
Jerk Seasoning /187
Mediteranean Seasoning /185
Taco Seasoning /188

STEP 3: CHOOSE YOUR VEGGIES

Something green and leafy: Lettuce, spinach, or kale.
A few colorful additions: Carrots, tomatoes, radishes.
Something to roast: Sweet potatoes, or Brussel sprouts.

ALWAYS PICK 2

When prepping for the week, choose 2 proteins that you can make at the same time. If you plan to bake, prep two sheet pans, each with a differently seasoned protein. Alternatively, plan on making one protein in your slow cooker or Instant pot, and one in the oven.

My favorite strategy is to make one pan of Chicken, seasoned with Mediterranean Seasoning and a second pan of Chicken with Taco Seasoning. Five minutes of prep, 20 minutes of baking time, and 2 minutes to clean up. That is only 7 minutes of hands-on time. You can do that!

PRO-TIP: Marinades freeze well, so plan to make a double batch anytime you marinade a protein. Toss one batch in the freezer for another week.

When shopping, I buy 4 ounces of meat for each serving that I need to make. Using this meathead math formula, one pound of protein will give you four servings. This is just a guideline to get you started. Some days I eat more or less, but this is a rough guideline. Adust as needed!

Download my Pick Two Guide from the blog at FoodologyGeek.com/BBN. Prep and then pack up your proteins. Store them in the refrigerator.

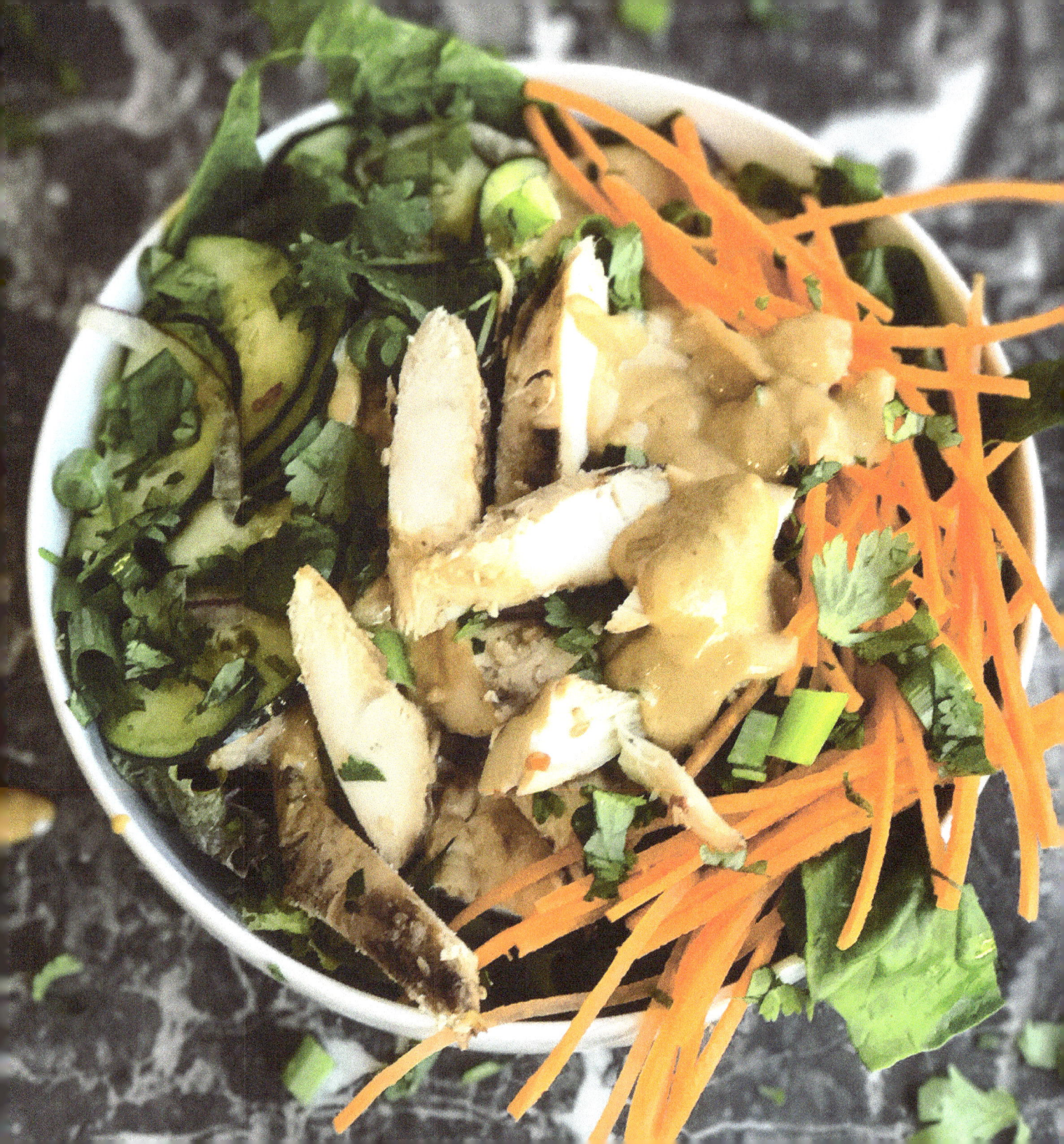

CHICKEN SATAY

MAKES 6 TO 8 SERVINGS

This Bowl is all about the sauce! You can slather the Peanut Satay Sauce on absolutely anything, and it's FANTASTIC! Crunchy-spicy cucumbers and marinated, grilled chicken full of umami – this Bowl a true winner. Go ahead, lick out the bowl, there's no judgment here!

You seriously can't get tired of eating this. The cucumber salad keeps well in the fridge and only gets better throughout the week, and the chicken is even tasty right out of the fridge.

INGREDIENTS

2 pounds chicken, breasts or thighs

SATAY MARINADE

¼ cup soy sauce or tamari
¼ cup rice wine vinegar
¼ cup water
2 tablespoons mirin
3 cloves garlic pressed
2 teaspoons fresh ginger grated
2 teaspoons crushed red pepper
2 teaspoons coconut oil
2 teaspoons yellow curry powder

FIXINS

Lettuce
Spinach
Shredded carrots
Green onions
Cilantro
Crushed Roasted Peanuts

EXTRAS

Asian Cucumber Salad /49
Satay Peanut Sauce /181

DIRECTIONS

Add all the ingredients to a gallon-sized freezer bag or a large nonreactive bowl and marinate for at least a few hours, up to overnight.

Remove the marinated chicken and place on a parchment-lined baking sheet.

Bake at 400°F for about 20 minutes.

NOTES

ALTERNATIVE: Place the chicken on skewers and grill for about 6 minutes on medium-high heat. This is my favorite way to cook them.

PALEO ADAPTABLE: Use almond butter instead of peanut butter.

VEGAN ADAPTABLE: Use seitan or pan-seared extra-firm tofu instead of chicken. Marinate the tofu for about 20 minutes before cooking it.

SHORTCUTS: Use frozen chicken tenderloins. If the chicken is still frozen, omit the water from the marinade.

Buy jars of minced garlic and grated ginger. These can usually be found in the produce section of the grocery store. You can also buy a teriyaki marinade and a sesame ginger salad dressing. Do what you can and don't sweat the rest. Baby steps!

PRO TIP: For super easy cleanup, I always line my baking sheet with parchment paper.

THE RIGHT TOOLS MAKE IT EASY

Like anything in life, having the right tools makes the job easier. You wouldn't try a DIY project without having the right tools. Meal prep is much easier to tackle if you have the tools you need and a plan to get you started.

BASIC KITCHEN TOOLS

- 6 Inch Chefs Knife
- Paring Knife
- 2 Rimmed Baking Sheets
- Skillet(s) 10 inch and 12 inch
- Dutch Oven
- Stock Pot
- 1 or 2 Sauce Pans
- 3 Large Bowls
- Pepper Grinder
- 7 to 14 Storage Containers
- Parchment Paper
- Cutting Board
- Kitchen Shears
- Peelers
- Rasp Grater
- Silicone Spatulas
- Tongs
- Measuring Tools
- Mandoline
- Spiralizer
- Meat Thermometer

ELECTRIC KITCHEN TOOLS

- Slow Cooker
- Instant Pot
- Pressure Cooker
- High Powered Blender
- Rice Cooker
- Electronic Probe Thermometer

Buy the items that you can afford and keep in mind that kitchen tools can last a lifetime, so invest wisely. Look for quality items that will hold up over time. Don't skimp on the tools that are going to help you live a healthier life.

I put together a whole page on the blog about my favorite kitchen tools. Some are absolutely necessary, and others are luxury items.

If you need more clarity about what to buy so that your kitchen is fully stocked and ready to rock meal prep, then head over to the blog and get my insider tips and helpful downloads.

You can shop for my favorite kitchen tools from my store at FoodologyGeek.com/BBN

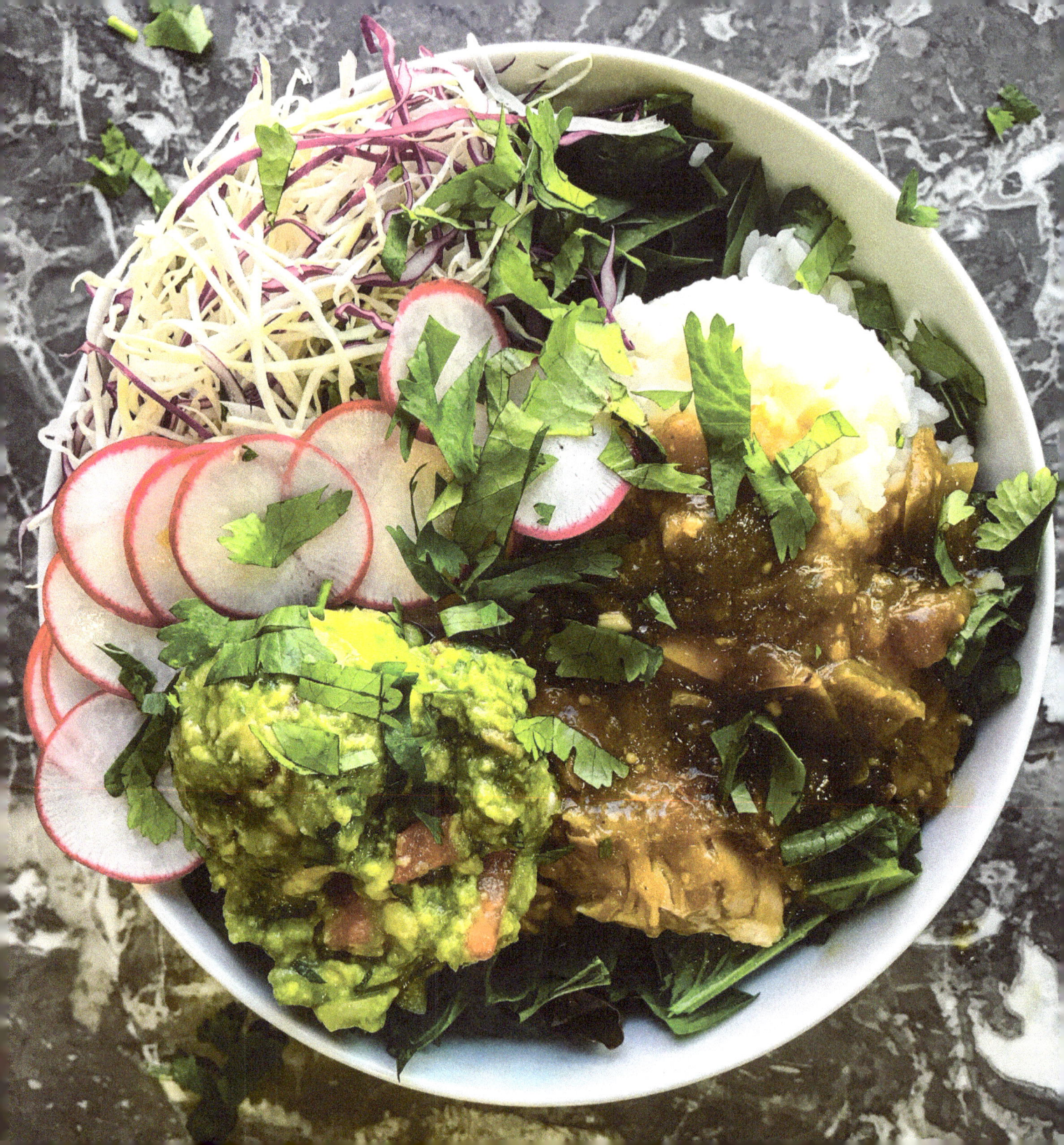

CHILI VERDE

MAKES 6 TO 8 SERVINGS

Chile Verde is one of my family's favorites, and this spicy green tomatillo sauce is incredibly flavorful and comforting. This recipe can be made with chicken, pork shoulder, heck, I even make it with tofu for my vegan daughter. Enjoy this spicy sauce on eggs, on rice, or on anything else you can put in your face.

INGREDIENTS

- 6 to 8 chicken breasts, bone-in or 3 to 4 pounds of pork shoulder.
- 1 tablespoon coconut oil
- 5 cloves garlic, minced
- ½ onion, diced
- 3 Anaheim chilis, seeded and diced
- 3 cans Hatch chilis, diced
- 2 pounds tomatillos, chopped and pureed
- 2 to 4 cups chicken broth, enough to cover the chicken
- ¼ bunch cilantro, diced

FIXINS

- Mexican Slaw or thinly sliced cabbage
- Radishes
- Cilantro
- Green onions

EXTRAS

Mexican Guacamole /67
Mexican Slaw /101

DIRECTIONS

Add the coconut oil, garlic, onion, and Anaheim chilis to a heavy-bottomed pot. Sauté until tender and fragrant.

Add the remaining ingredients.

Make sure that there's enough liquid to cover the meat.

Bring everything to a boil, then reduce to a simmer.

Cover and simmer 30 to 40 minutes. There should be a small amount of liquid covering the meat at all times.

When the chicken is tender, remove it from the heat and let it cool slightly.

Pull the chicken out of the sauce and remove the bones. Chop up the chicken and then return the chopped chicken to the pot.

NOTES

SHORTCUTS: Substitute a 28-ounce can of green enchilada sauce instead of tomatillos. You can also use diced boneless chicken breasts to bring the cooking time down to 20 minutes.

PRO TIP: Use a slow cooker or Instant Pot to cook up this green chili.

VEGAN ADAPTABLE: I've made this many times with extra-firm tofu, and it tastes great. One of the things I do when I am cooking for my vegan daughter is that before I add any protein to the Chili Verde, I ladle out a portion for her and set it aside in a small saucepan. Then I add the diced tofu to hers and the chicken or pork to ours.

MEAL PREP ALTERNATIVES

MAKE SOUP: To make the Chili Verde into a hearty soup, just add a little extra water or broth to it. I love eating this soup version with a little sour cream or crème fraiche and some fresh cilantro on top.

FREEZE: Chili Verde freezes really well. Keep in the freezer for 4-6 months.

LEFTOVERS: Once we have eaten all the meat out of it, I use the remaining Chili Verde as a sauce on tacos or eggs.

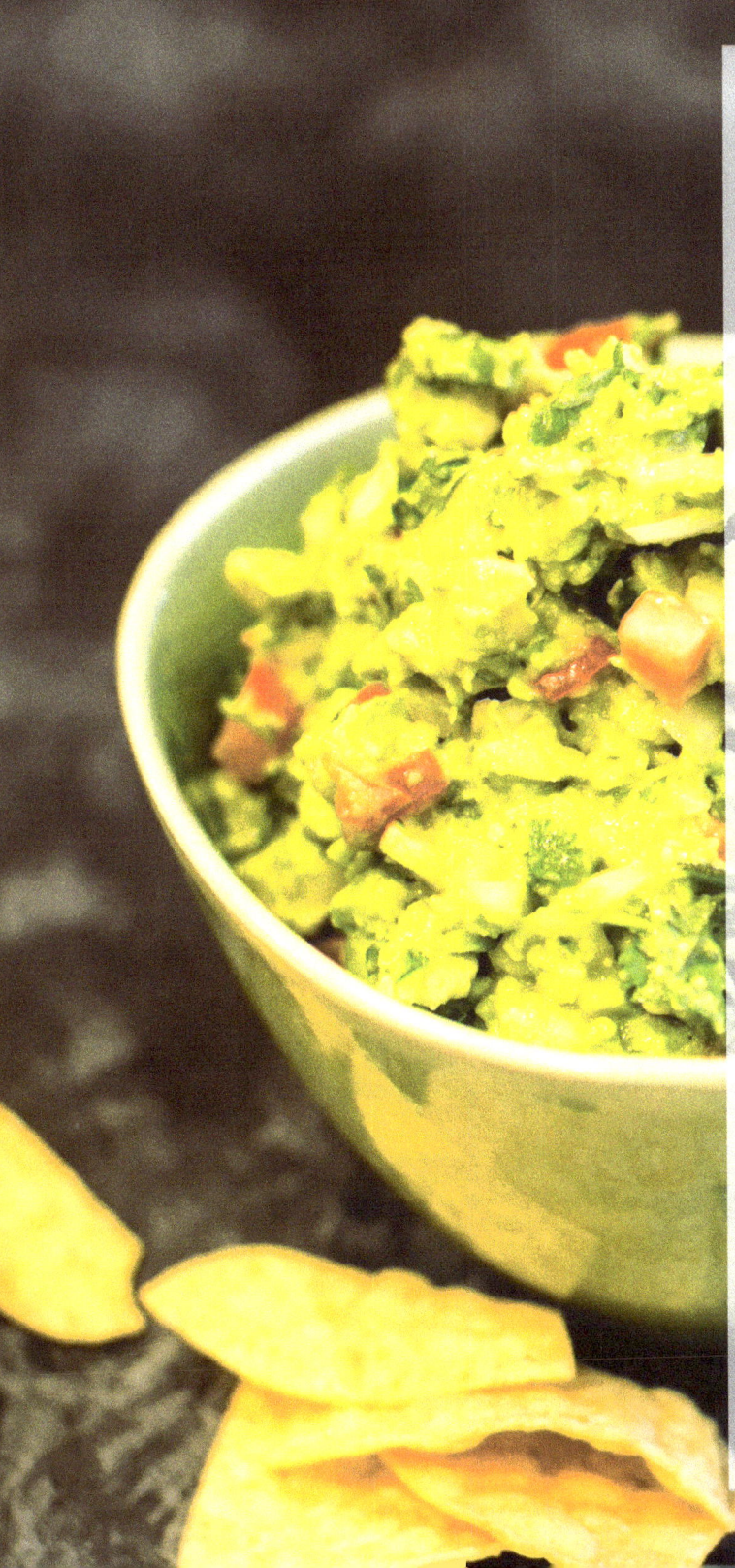

MEXICAN GUACAMOLE

INGREDIENTS

4 avocados
½ white onion, finely diced
2 limes, juiced
2 teaspoons Kosher salt
¼ teaspoon black pepper
½ bunch cilantro, finely diced
2 jalapeños or serrano peppers, finely diced
¾ cup fresh tomatoes, finely diced

DIRECTIONS

Halve the avocados and scoop out the flesh.

Use a fork to mash the avocados until they are smooth but still a little bit chunky.

Add the onions, lime, salt, and pepper. Taste and adjust the salt and lime if needed.

Add the cilantro, jalapeños, and tomatoes, if using.

Store any leftovers in an airtight container in the refrigerator.

NOTES

PRO TIPS: Use tomatoes only if they are in season and really ripe. Mix them in just prior to serving. You can also substitute a few tablespoons of Salsa Fresca /72

When storing leftover guacamole, press plastic wrap onto the surface to seal out any air. Another handy tip is to put the pit back into the guacamole before you store it.

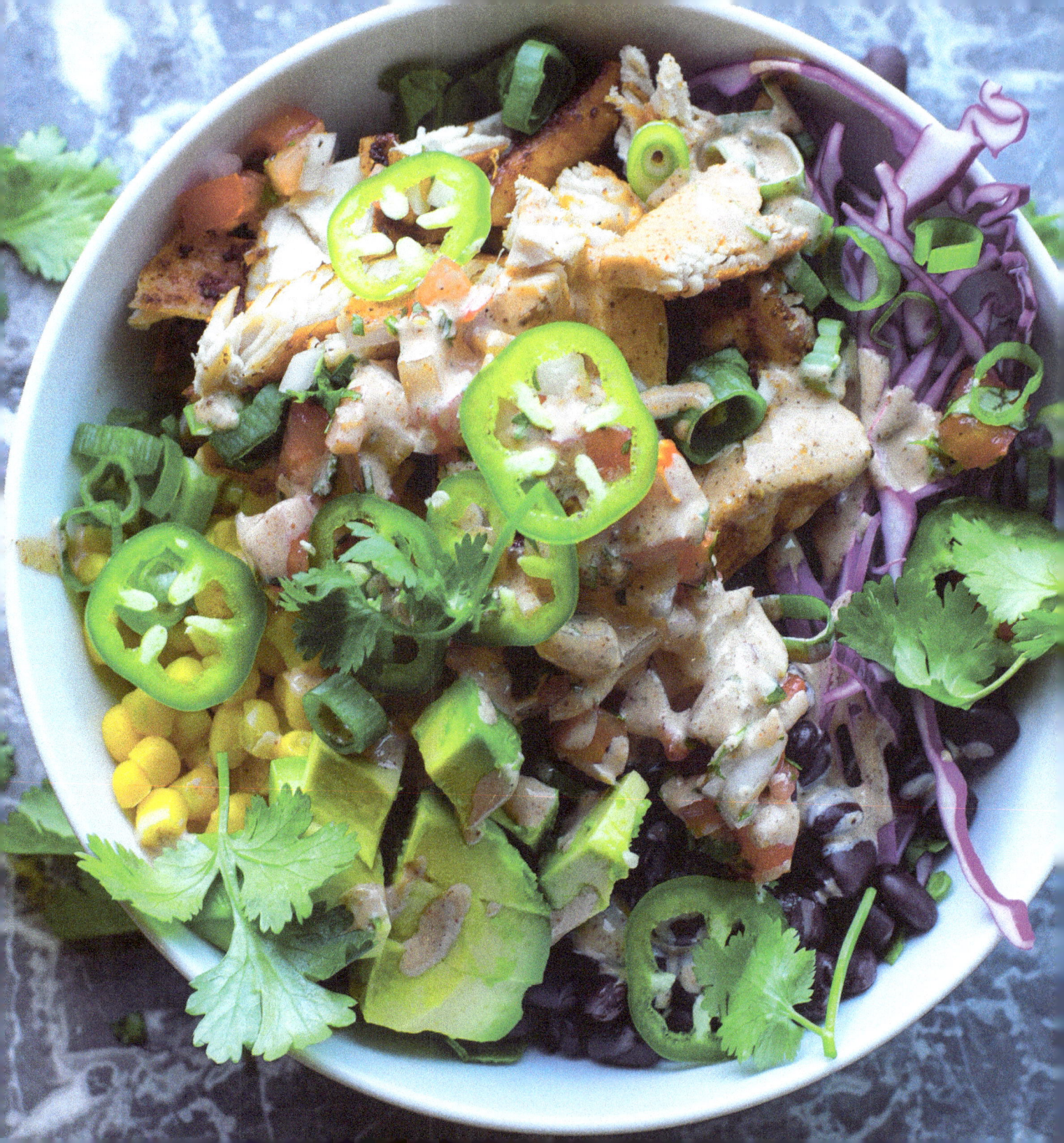

CHIPOTLE CHICKEN

MAKES 6 TO 8 SERVINGS

Imagine the best chicken burrito you've ever had, and then just put it in a bowl! Why go out to eat when you can make this in less time? With just 10 minutes of prep and 10 minutes of cooking, this is faster, cheaper, and (of course) healthier than heading out to buy a burrito bowl! Plus, with the leftovers, you can just put this on repeat all week!

INGREDIENTS

2 pounds chicken, breasts or thighs
2 teaspoons avocado oil or coconut oil
2 tablespoons Taco Seasoning Mix /188

FIXINS

Romaine lettuce
Spinach
Red cabbage
Corn, fresh or frozen
Black beans
Green onions
Avocados
Jalapeños
Cilantro

EXTRAS

Mexican Guacamole /67
Mexican Slaw /101
Roasted Corn Salsa /71
Chipotle Ranch /157
Roasted Sweet Potatoes /131
Salsa Fresca /72

DIRECTIONS

Preheat the oven to 425°F.

Toss the meat with salt, pepper, taco seasoning and a little avocado or coconut oil.

Bake for 15 to 20 minutes.

Rest for 5 to 10 minutes and chop.

NOTES

STOVE TOP: Dice and pan sauté over medium-high heat for 6 to 10 minutes.

ALTERNATIVE: Use pork, beef, fish, or shrimp.

VEGAN ADAPTABLE: Leave out the meat altogether.

PRO TIPS: If you're making the Roasted Southwest Sweet Potatoes, make sure these go in the oven at the same time as the chicken. They can even go on the same pan if you have room.

You will use the Taco Seasoning Mix in the Chipotle Ranch and the Roasted Southwest Sweet Potatoes. You'll also have leftover Taco Seasoning Mix. Save it for next time.

SHORTCUT: Use pre-made taco seasoning.

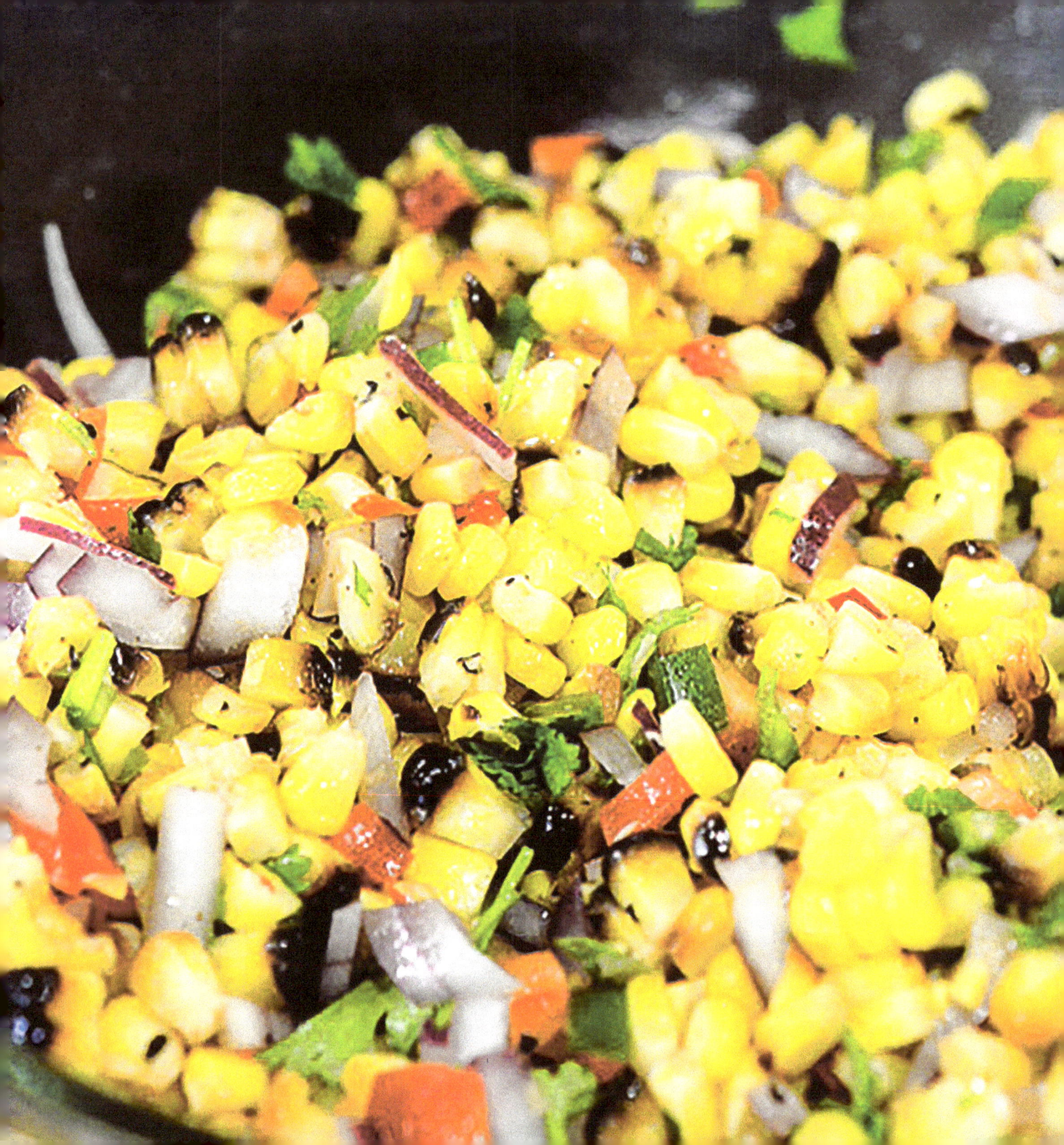

ROASTED CORN SALSA

INGREDIENTS

2 ears fresh corn
1 red bell pepper, finely diced
2 jalapeños or serrano peppers, finely diced
½ red onion, finely diced
⅓ bunch cilantro, finely chopped
1 teaspoon cumin
1 teaspoon Kosher salt
¼ teaspoon black pepper
1 lime, juiced
2 teaspoons olive oil or avocado oil

DIRECTIONS

Oven roast or grill the corn on the cob.

Let the corn cool. Once cool, cut the kernels from the cob. Place the kernels in a large nonreactive bowl.

Dice and chop all the vegetables and add them to the bowl.

Add cumin, lime juice, olive oil, and salt and pepper to taste.

Toss all the ingredients together. Store any leftovers in an airtight container in the refrigerator.

NOTES

OVEN ROASTING: Remove the husks. Roast the corn on a broiler pan, rotating the corn as it starts to get charred. The oven rack should be close to the top of the oven, about 6 to 8 inches from the heat source.

GRILLING: Leave the husks on the corn. Place the corn directly on the grill. Grill until the kernels inside are well browned and charred in places.

SHORTCUT: Use frozen corn. Cook it according to the package directions and let cool before adding it to the salsa.

SALSA FRESCA

INGREDIENTS

4 cups tomatoes, chopped
2 jalapeños, finely diced
2 serrano peppers, finely diced
2 cloves garlic, minced or pressed
½ white onion, diced
½ bunch cilantro, finely chopped
1 small cucumber, finely diced (optional)
1 lime, juiced
2 teaspoons olive oil
2 teaspoons Kosher salt
1 teaspoon black pepper

DIRECTIONS

Dice and chop all the vegetables and add them to a large nonreactive bowl.

Add lime juice, olive oil, and salt and pepper to taste. Toss to combine.

Store in an airtight container in the refrigerator.

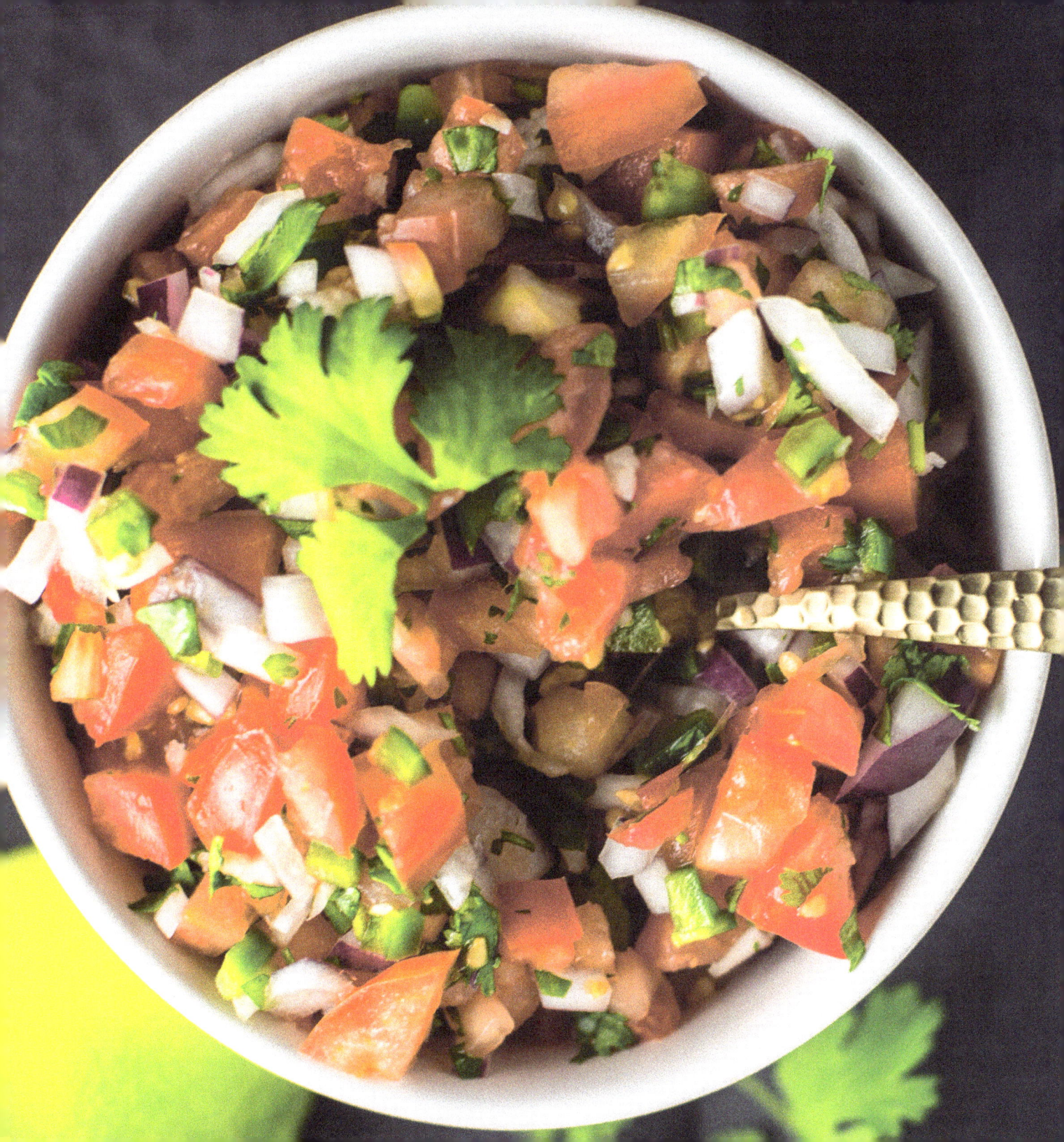

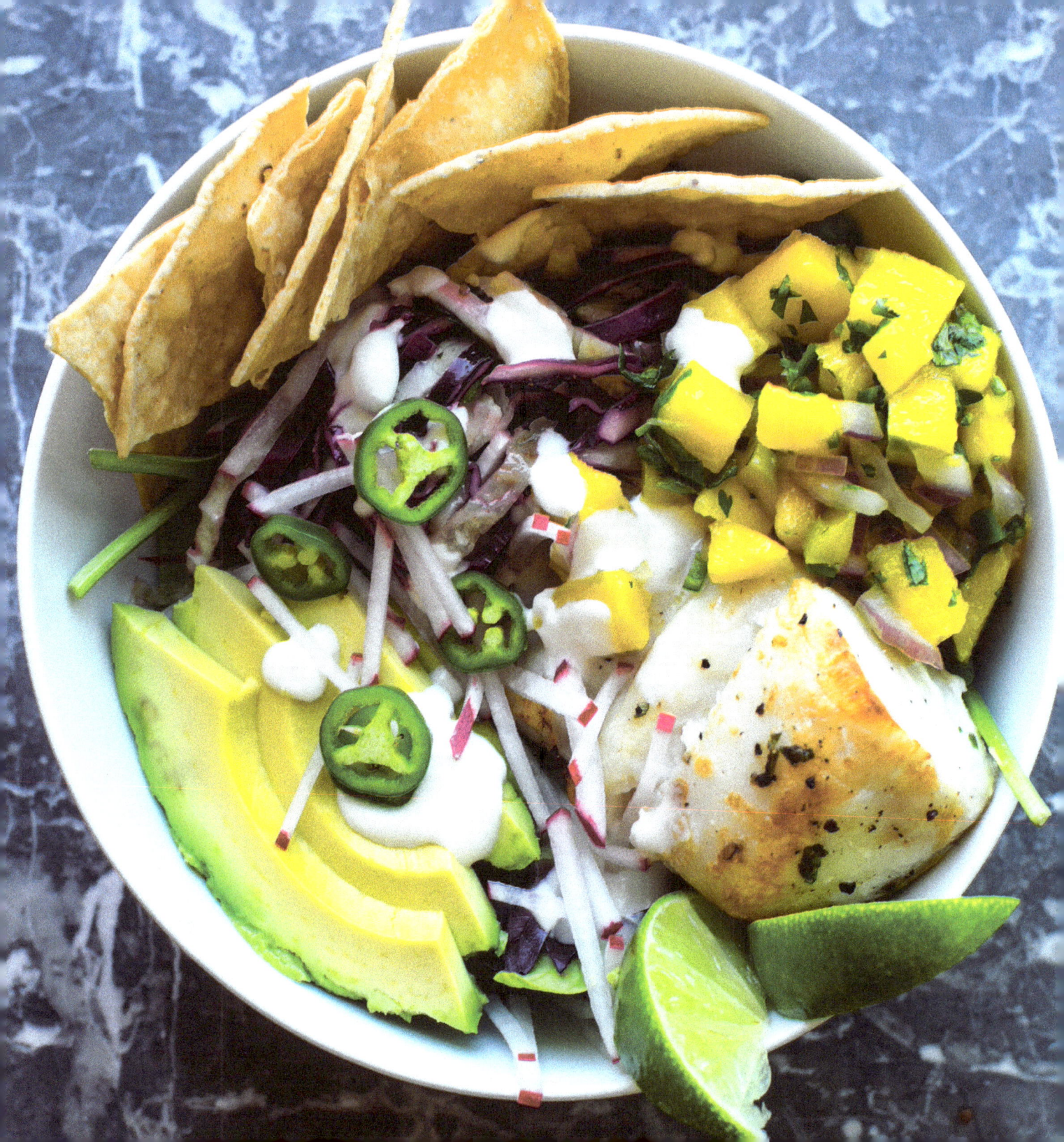

TEQUILA LIME FISH

MAKES 6 TO 8 SERVINGS

When I lived in San Diego, a stone's throw from Baja California, I became a big fan of the fish taco. This Bowl's inspiration lies in memories that I cherish: my many trips to Baja in search of good surf and food, and my mom's tequila lime chicken pasta recipe. I've combined these two fantastic flavors to create a healthy flavor bomb of a bowl.

INGREDIENTS

2 pounds of cod, cut into 6 to 8 fillets

TEQUILA LIME MARINADE

1 shot tequila
1 tablespoon avocado oil or coconut oil
½ lime, juiced
1 tablespoon cilantro, minced
½ teaspoon Kosher salt
¼ teaspoon black pepper

FIXINS

2 avocados or 1 container of prepared guacamole
4 radishes, julienned
8 cups mixed greens
Fresh jalapeños or serrano peppers
Limes for squeezing

EXTRAS

Mexican Guacamole /67
Mexican Slaw /101
Mango Salsa /77

DIRECTIONS

Add all of the ingredients to a gallon-sized freezer bag or a large nonreactive bowl, marinate at least 20 minutes, up to a few hours.

Remove the fish from the marinade and place it on a parchment lined baking sheet.

Broil until the fish is slightly brown and firm to touch, 8 to 10 minutes.

Let the fish rest for about 5 minutes before serving.

NOTES

ALTERNATIVE: Use chicken or shrimp.

VEGAN ADAPTABLE: Use extra-firm tofu and chickpeas. Bake or pan sear after marinating.

CHOOSING FISH: Almost all seafood that you buy in the grocery store has been previously frozen and then thawed so that it can be displayed in the case. For this reason, I usually buy my fish frozen and pre-portioned. It makes meal prep a breeze, and it also allows me to have fish in the freezer to cook any time I need a quick meal. Try to buy fish from sustainable sources whenever possible.

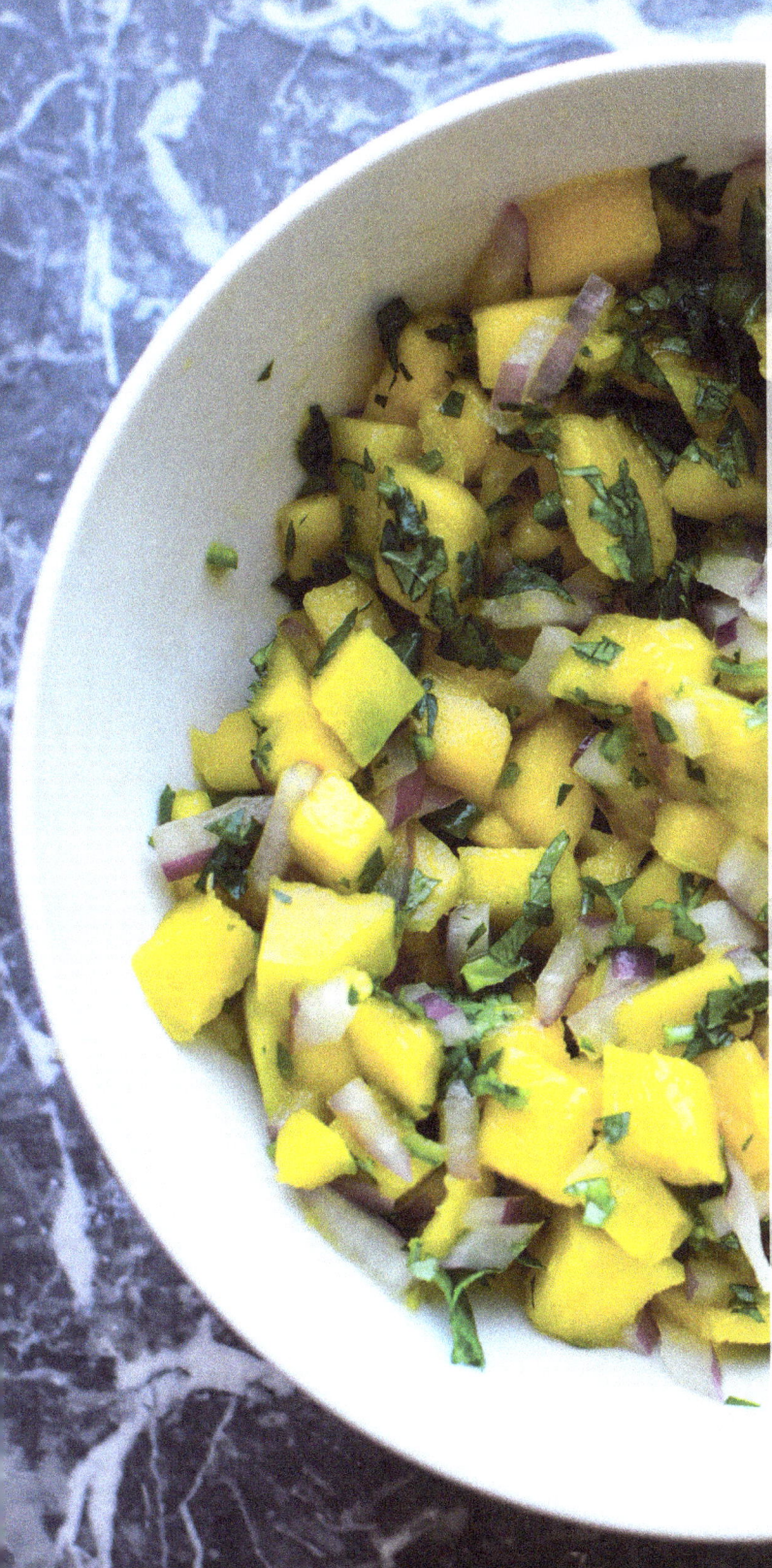

MANGO SALSA

INGREDIENTS

1 mango, diced
1 jalapeño, minced
¼ red onion, finely diced
2 tablespoons cilantro, finely minced
½ lime, juiced
1 teaspoon avocado oil
½ teaspoon Kosher salt

DIRECTIONS

Dice and chop all the fruits and vegetables.

Toss in a large nonreactive bowl.

Add lime juice, avocado oil, and salt to taste. Toss.

Store any leftovers in an airtight container in the refrigerator.

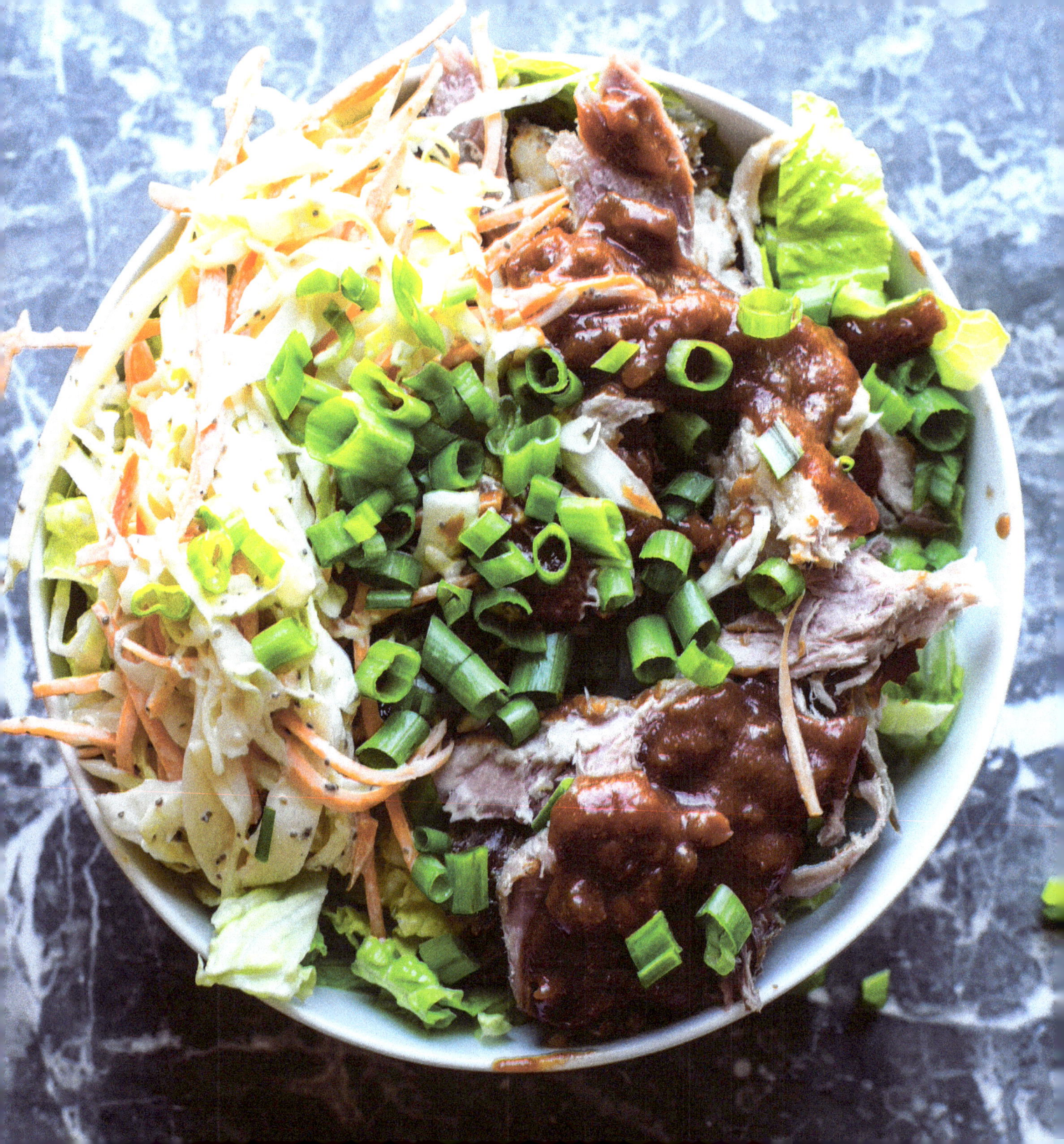

BARBECUE PULLED PORK

MAKES 12 TO 16 SERVINGS

This rich and meaty barbecue pulled pork is super easy to prepare using a slow cooker or Instant Pot. Turn this meat into something Beast Bowl-worthy by smothering it with delicious Spicy Tangy Barbecue Sauce and then topping it with a healthy helping of crunchy, creamy Southern Coleslaw.

INGREDIENTS

4 pounds pork shoulder

2 to 3 tablespoons Barbecue Spice Rub /187

FIXINS

Green onions

Romaine lettuce

Spinach

EXTRAS

Southern Coleslaw /80

Spicy Tangy Barbecue Sauce /173

MEAL PREP ALTERNATIVES

MAKE TACOS: This is always a go-to when I have leftovers. Shredded pork tacos are delicious.

MAKE LETTUCE WRAPS: Add some shredded pork to a lettuce cup and top it with matchstick veggies. (You can buy these pre-prepped.) Finish it with a little of your favorite dressing.

DIRECTIONS

Make the Barbecue Spice Rub.

Rub the pork shoulder with 4 to 5 tablespoons of the spice rub.

Put the pork shoulder in the slow cooker, fattiest side up. Do not add any liquid.

Cook until the meat is tender and falling apart, about 3 to 4 hours on high depending on the size of your roast.

Remove the meat from the slow cooker, let it rest for about 20 minutes, and then shred it with forks.

NOTES

SUBSTITUTIONS: You can use chicken instead of pork. If you have some barbecue expertise, try brisket.

VEGAN ADAPTABLE: Use jackfruit, fresh or canned.

PRO TIP: Leave the slow cooker on high only if you will be home. Leave it on low if you will be out all day. If you are leaving the roast for more than 8 hours, add about 1 cup of water to make sure you still have moisture in the slow cooker. If you're using an Instant Pot, follow the directions for your kitchen appliance.

SHORTCUT: Find a bottled barbecue sauce and skip making your own.

BEAST BOWL NUTRITION | CHAPTER 4 | CORE PROTEINS & EXTRAS

SOUTHERN COLESLAW

INGREDIENTS

1 cup carrots, shredded
4 cups cabbage, finely shredded
4 to 6 green onions, sliced

COLESLAW DRESSING

2 tablespoons onion, grated
½ cup avocado mayonnaise
1 tablespoon Dijon mustard
1 tablespoon apple cider vinegar
3 teaspoons granulated sugar
1 teaspoon Kosher salt
½ teaspoon celery salt
1 teaspoon celery seed

DIRECTIONS

Shred the carrots and cabbage and add them to a large bowl.

Add all the dressing ingredients to a medium bowl and whisk.

Use ½ cup of dressing. (You will have dressing left over.)

Toss and let the slaw set in the refrigerator for an hour before serving. Garnish with green onions.

Store any leftovers in an airtight container in the refrigerator.

NOTES

SHORTCUT: Use prepackaged coleslaw mix from your produce section and buy your coleslaw dressing. Even easier, buy your coleslaw already prepared from the deli!

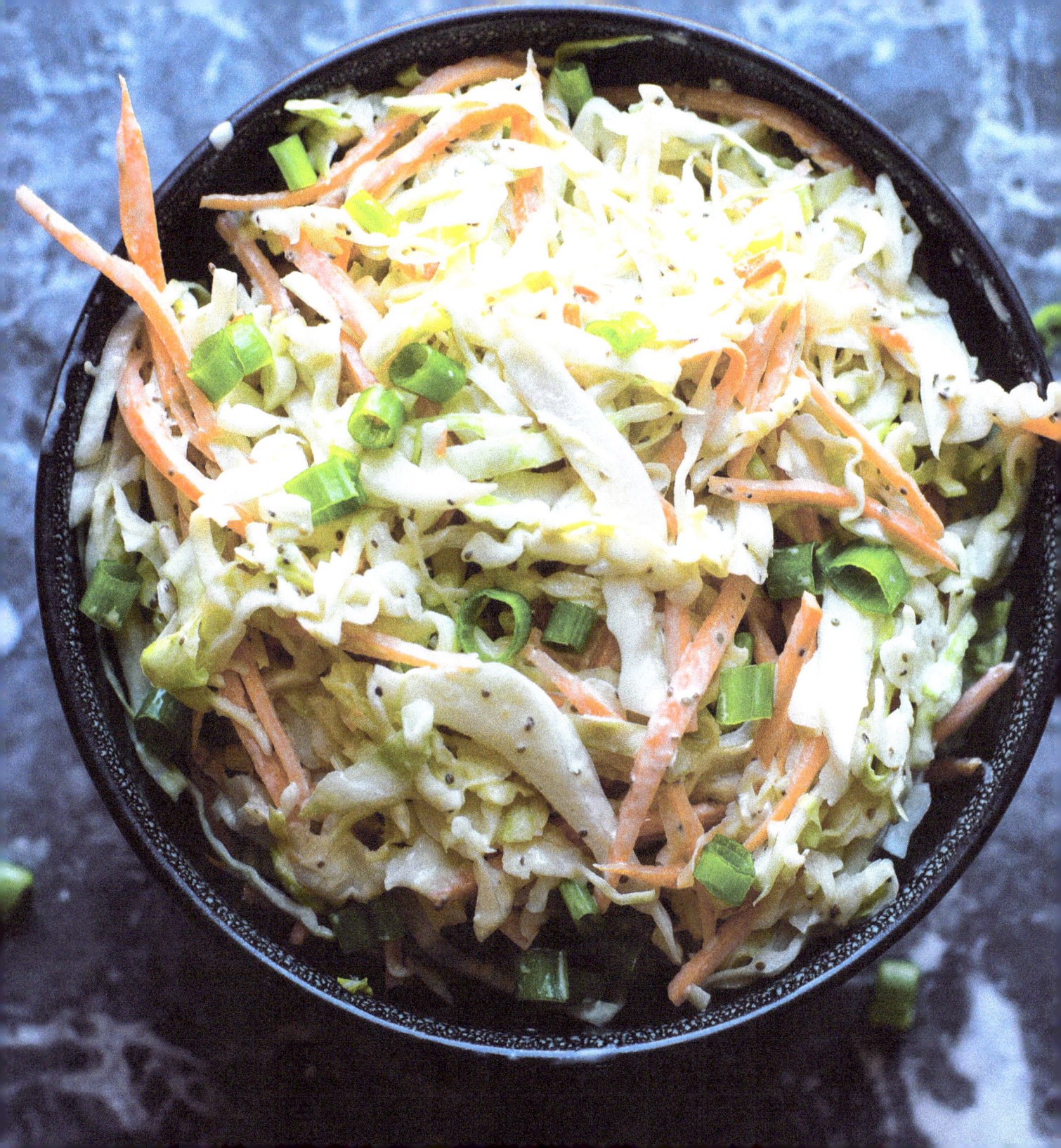

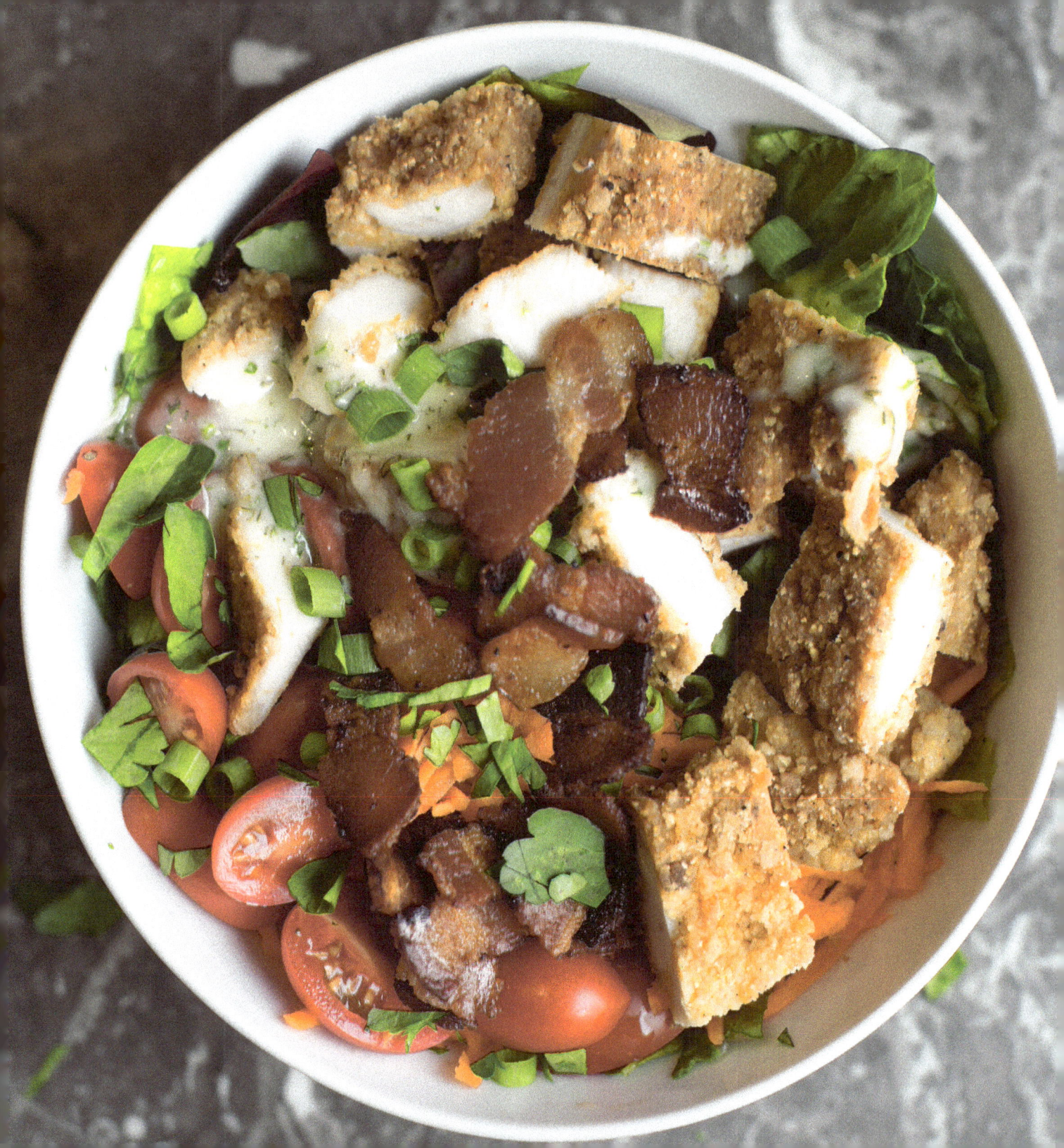

FRIED CHICKEN

MAKES 6 TO 8 SERVINGS

Everybody needs some fried chicken in their life! This recipe is gluten-free, but you can also make it using regular flour if you don't have an issue with gluten. Brining the chicken before you fry it makes it extra juicy. Not only is this chicken fantastic and super flavorful, but the crust is crispy and stays put on the meat.

INGREDIENTS

1 pound bacon, fried; grease reserved.
3 pounds boneless chicken, breasts or thighs
Oil for frying, avocado oil or other high heat oil

BUTTERMILK MARINADE

2 cups buttermilk, or 1 15-ounce can coconut milk
2 eggs
1 teaspoon paprika
1 teaspoon onion powder
2 teaspoons Kosher salt
½ teaspoon cayenne pepper
½ teaspoon black pepper

BREADING

1½ cups gluten-free flour blend
½ cup cornmeal
¼ cup cornstarch
1 teaspoon baking soda
1 teaspoon onion powder
1 teaspoon paprika
2 teaspoons Kosher salt
½ teaspoon black pepper
½ teaspoon cayenne pepper

FIXINS

Lettuce
Spinach
Shredded carrots
Tomatoes
Bacon crumbles
Green onions

EXTRAS

Paleo Ranch /155

DIRECTIONS

Add all the marinade ingredients to a gallon-sized freezer bag or a large nonreactive bowl.

Cut the chicken into chicken finger sized pieces.

Marinate the chicken for a few hours at room temperature. You can also refrigerate the marinating chicken for up to 2 days before cooking.

Dice the bacon and fry it on medium-low heat until crispy.

Remove the bacon and set it aside.

Reserve the bacon grease for frying the chicken tenders. Alternatively, use another type of oil.

PRO TIP: You may need extra oil. Schmaltz, which is rendered chicken fat, is the absolute most perfect frying fat for this recipe. If you can't find this at your local market, you should be able to find it online. Check out my shop of ingredients at FoodologyGeek.com/BBN

Prepare a baking sheet and set a cooling rack over the top.

Add all the dry ingredients to a shallow bowl for dredging the chicken tenders.

Dredge each chicken tender and then set them aside on the sheet pan.

Heat the frying grease or oil to 350°F. Use a thermometer to make sure the temperature stays between 300°F and 325°F during cooking.

The chicken tenders will fry for 2 to 3 minutes on each side, depending on the temperature of the oil.

When the chicken tenders are nicely browned, remove them from the oil and set them on a cooling rack.

NOTES

Bring refrigerated chicken to room temperature by leaving it on the counter for about 30 minutes before cooking.

THE SCIENCE OF FAT

Fat is an essential part of making food tasty and satiating. Find the skinny on fat and oil by downloading my Definitive Cooking Oil and Fat Guide. Find it at FoodologyGeek.com/BBN

UNSATURATED FATS

Monounsaturated and polyunsaturated fats are liquid at room temperature and usually solid when refrigerated. These oils are derived from nuts and olives. Walnut oil, olive oil, avocado oil are all great examples of monounsaturated fats.

Avocado oil is my favorite oil to cook with. It is flavorful in dressings and has a high smoke point so it works well for searing meat too! It's a flavorful multitasker.

SATURATED FATS

Saturated fat is solid at room temperature because it is saturated with Hydrogens. Naturally, saturated fats include animal fats, such as lard, suet, and schmaltz. I like to use rendered fat for cooking. Other notable saturated fats include butter, ghee, and fat found in dairy. Palm and coconut oil are also saturated fats.

At one time, saturated fats had a bad reputation. However, current research has shown them to be anti-inflammatory. They do not contain trans fats. Saturated fats are also best for cooking at high heats.

HYDROGENATED FATS

Hydrogenation is a chemical process that turns a liquid vegetable fat into a solid vegetable fat by adding hydrogens. Enter shortening! The hydrogenation process produces trans fats. Commercially produced lard is also hydrogenated.

Processed foods contain a high amount of hydrogenated oils and these trans fats. Hydrogenated oils cause inflammation and lead to many serious health issues.

THE 411 ON OIL

SATURATED FATS

Butter
Ghee
Lard (non-hydrogenated)
Suet
Shamltz

UNSATURATED FATS

Avocado Oil
Canola Oil
Coconut Oil
Corn Oil
Nut Oil
Olive Oil
Peanut Oil
Safflower Oil
Soybean Oil
Sunflower Oil
Vegetable Oil Blend

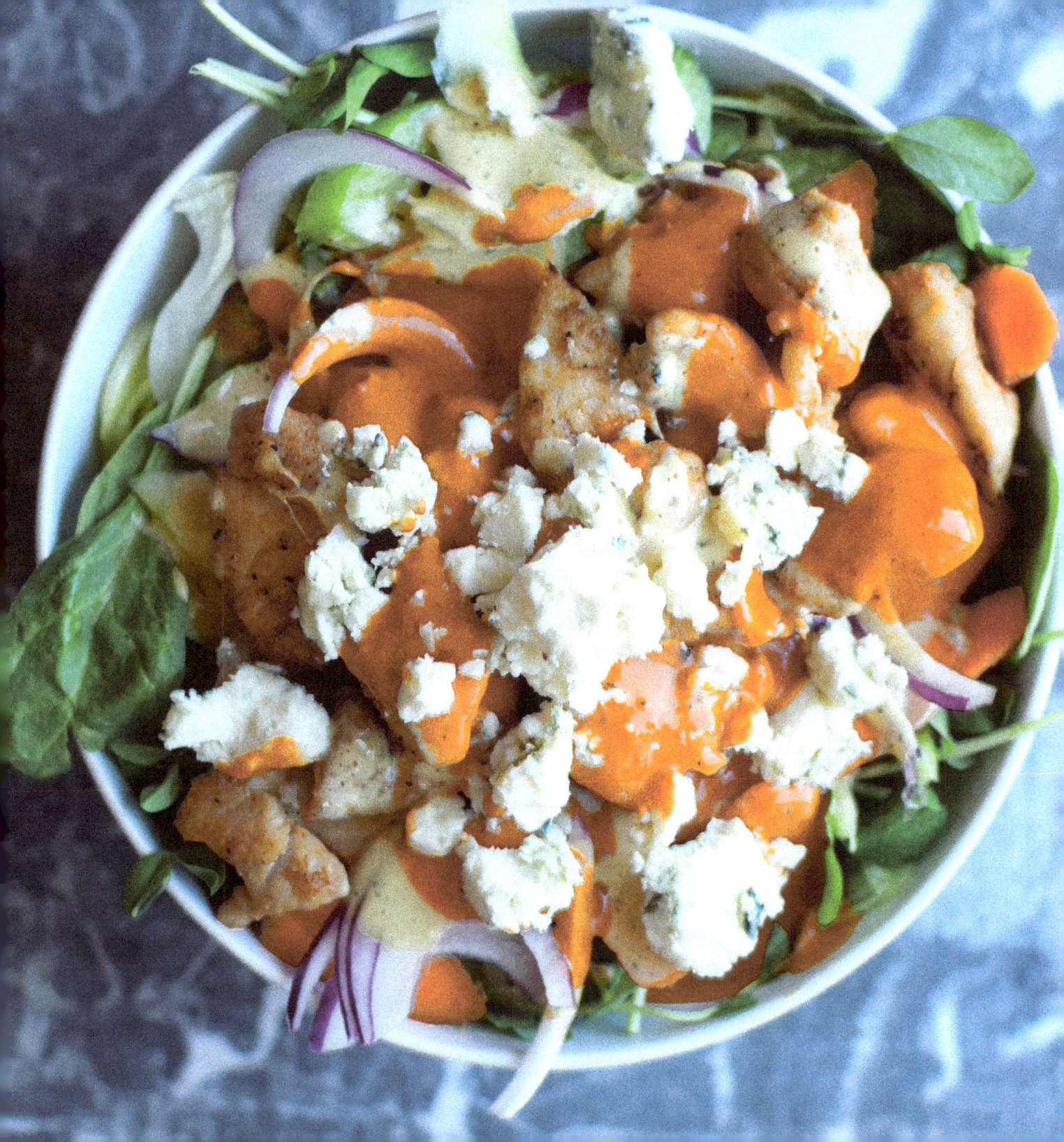

BUFFALO CHICKEN

MAKES 6 TO 8 SERVINGS

This Bowl is made up of all of the goodness you get with a basket of hot wings… the celery and carrots, a little ranch, and some blue cheese. I whip up a fast and tasty Buffalo Ranch and top it with some crumbled blue cheese. This Bowl has everything in it to satisfy your craving for hot wings while still keeping you on track for healthy eating.

Ditch the deep-fried wings and chow down on this Beast Bowl instead! No regrets here!

INGREDIENTS

- 2 to 3 pounds chicken, breasts or thighs
- 2 teaspoons of coconut oil
- 1 tablespoon Buffalo Seasoning Mix /186

FIXINS

- Blue cheese
- Buffalo wing sauce
- Romaine lettuce
- Spinach
- Microgreens
- Carrots
- Celery
- Red onions

EXTRAS

- Buffalo Ranch /156

DIRECTIONS

Dice the thawed chicken into bite-sized pieces and sprinkle with the Buffalo Seasoning Mix.

Add a few teaspoons of coconut oil to a skillet on medium-high heat.

Sauté until lightly browned.

NOTES

ALTERNATIVE: Use shrimp instead of chicken.

SHORTCUT: Use frozen chicken tenderloins. Thaw before baking.

PRO TIP: Make a big batch of seasoning mix so you can easily make this chicken any time.

BAKE: Bake at 400°F for about 20 minutes on a parchment-lined baking sheet.

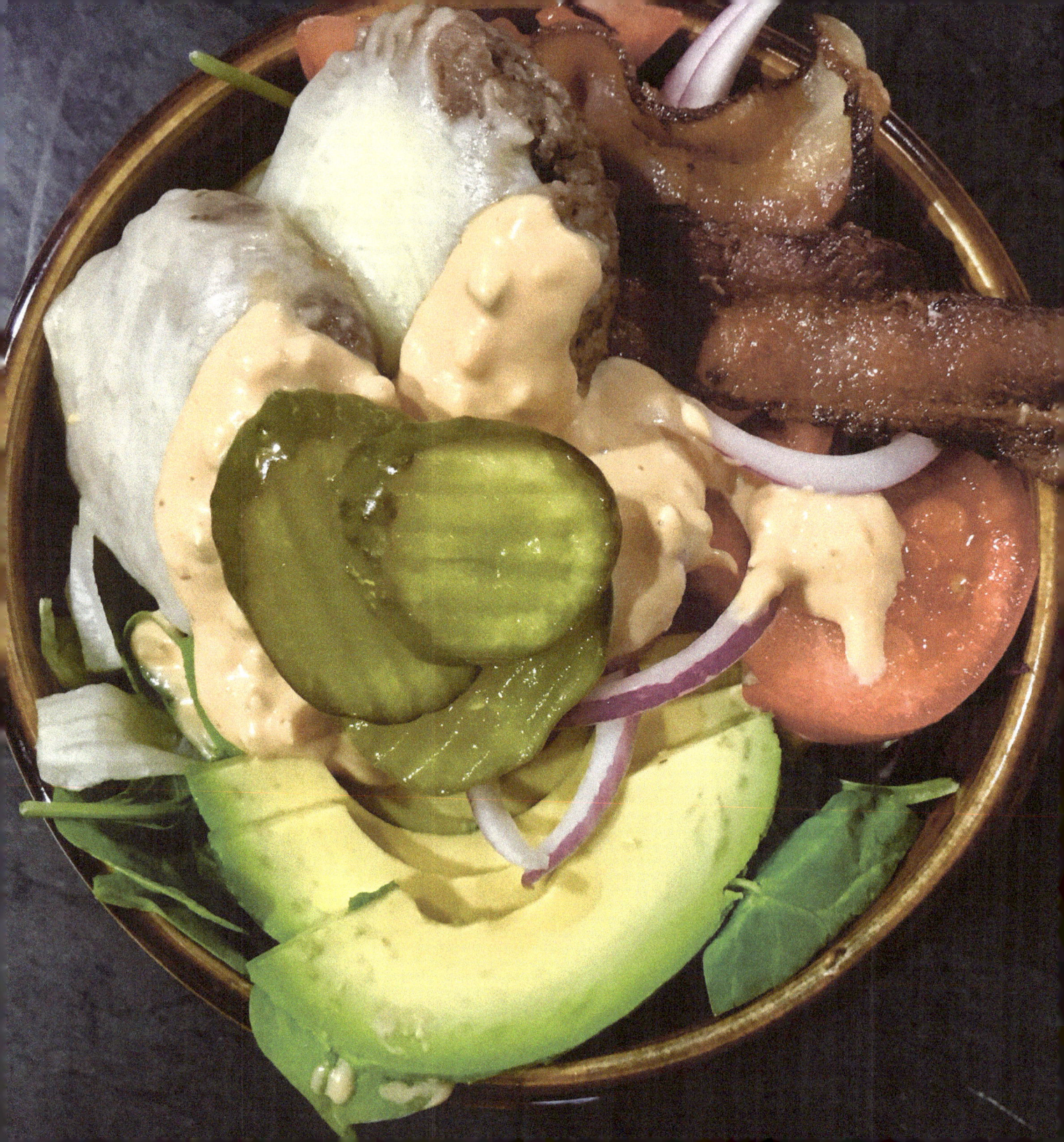

ALL-AMERICAN BURGER

MAKES 8 TO 12 SERVINGS

Get all the mayhem of a legit Beast-style burger, complete with some sloppy, tasty Beast Sauce, but minus all the guilt! Dial things up with some bacon and avocado, and if you're ready to go ALL IN and make it a cheeseburger situation, add your favorite cheese to these mini burgers.

Have room for extra carbs? Add some oven-baked fries.

INGREDIENTS

2 to 3 pounds grass-fed ground beef
Kosher salt
Black pepper
Cheese (optional)

BEAST SAUCE

⅓ cup mayonnaise
¼ cup ketchup
1½ tablespoons yellow mustard
¼ cup sweet pickle relish

Whisk all the ingredients together.

Store any leftovers in an airtight container in the refrigerator.

FIXINS

Avocados
Bacon
Cheese
Dill pickles
Iceberg lettuce
Spinach
Tomatoes
Red onion

EXTRAS

Oven Roasted Potatoes /129
Beastastic Mayo /153
Paleo Ketchup /167

DIRECTIONS

Add salt and pepper to the meat.

Mix well with your hands.

Divide the meat into 8 small burger patties.

Fry or grill the patties on medium-high for about 3 minutes each side.

If you're using cheese, add the cheese in the last 30 seconds.

Remove the burgers from heat and place them on a plate.

Let the burgers rest for about 10 minutes, covered loosely with foil, while you prepare the rest of the bowl.

NOTES

VEGAN ADAPTABLE: Use veggie burgers and vegan mayo.

PRO TIP: Use a large cookie scoop for perfect portions every time.

MEAL PREP ALTERNATIVES FOR LEFTOVERS

MAKE TACOS: Leftover burgers can be chopped up and warmed up with some taco seasoning. This repurposing of the ground beef can be used for your own Taco Tuesday or used to make a different Beast Bowl, like the Mom-Style Taco Bowl.

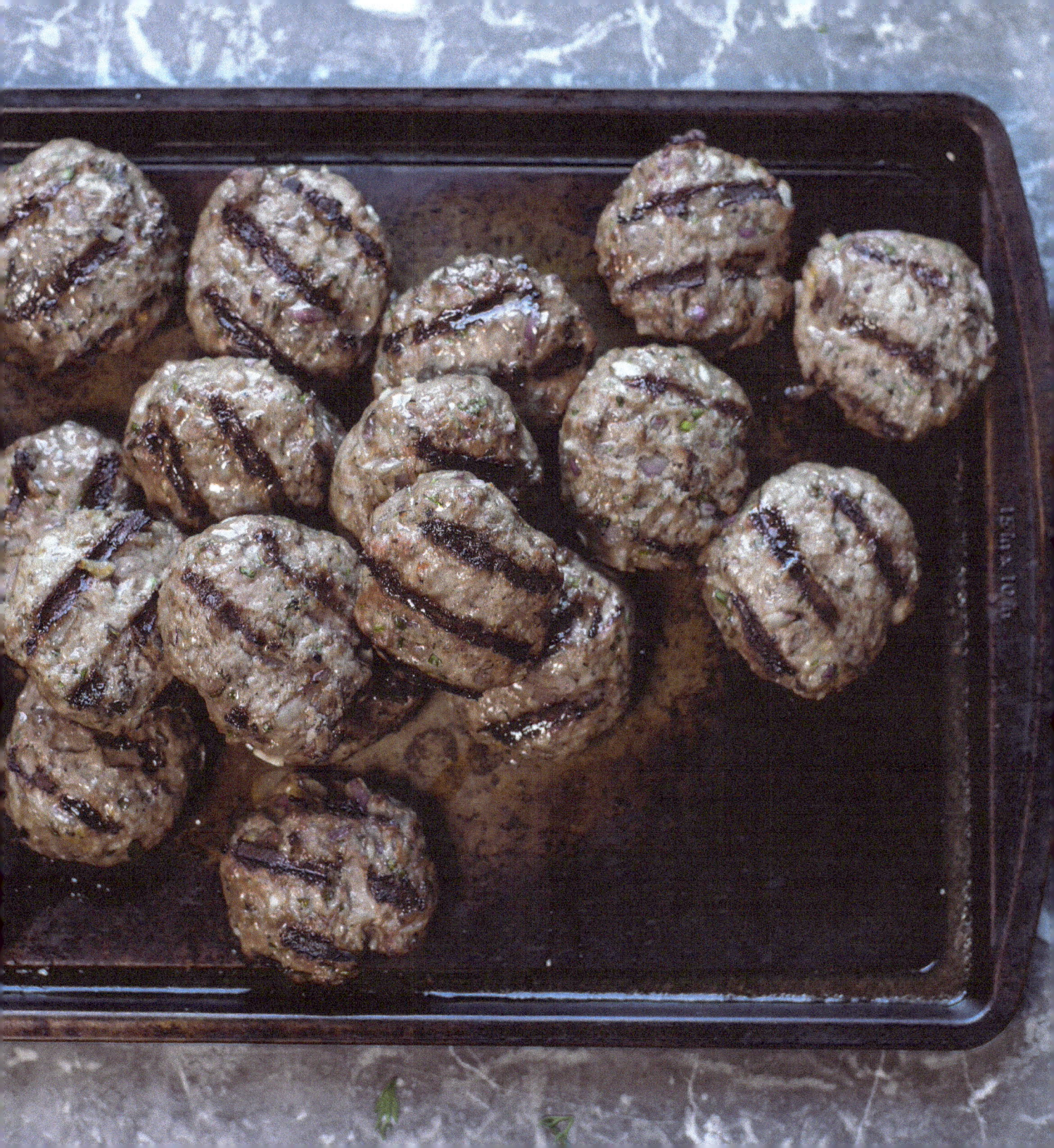

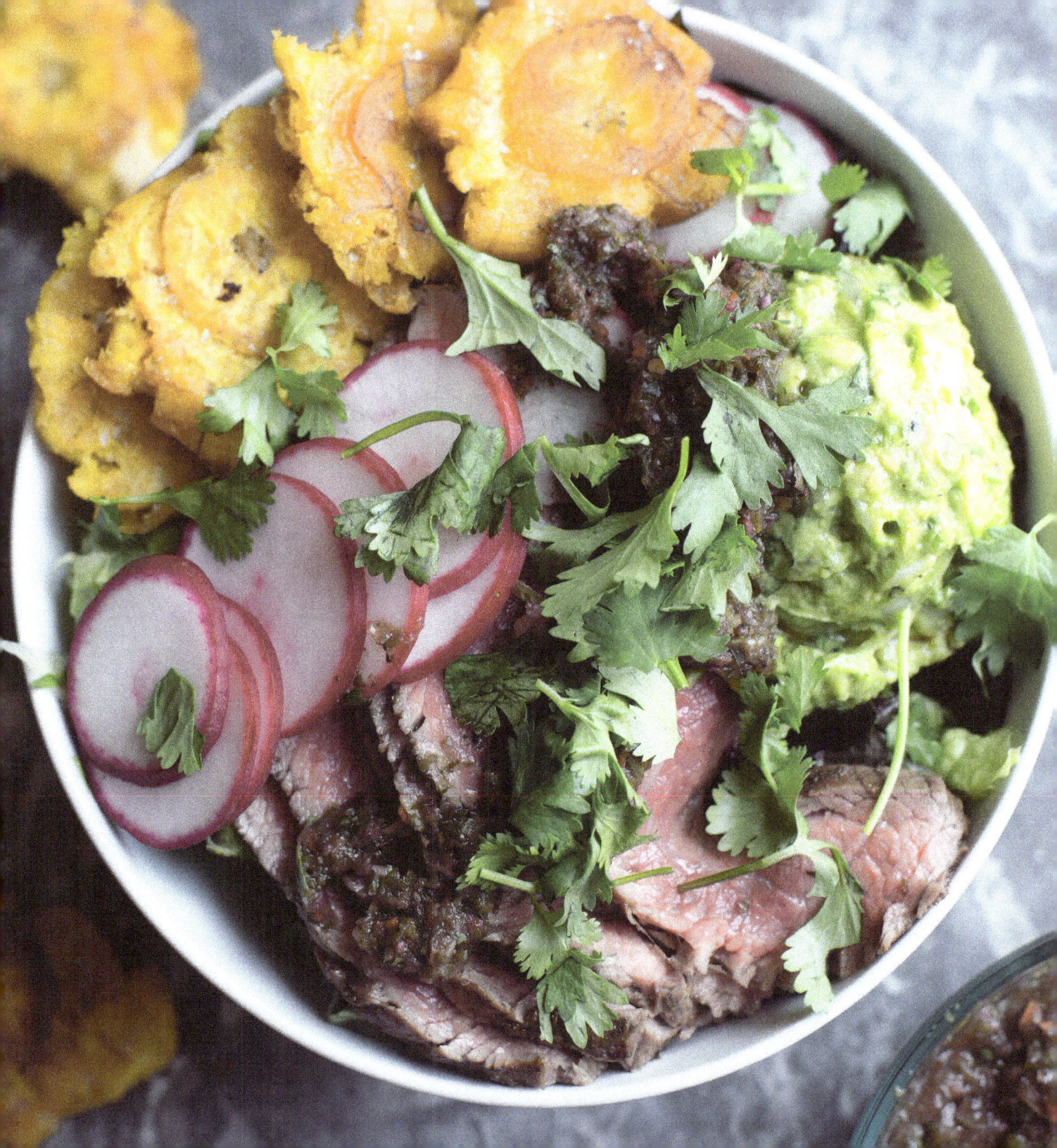

STEAK CHIMICHURRI

MAKES 6 TO 8 SERVINGS

Overcome any meal prep boredom you may have with this spicy, protein-packed Steak Chimichurri Beast Bowl!

There are three reasons why this Bowl checks all the boxes. One: grilled marinated hanger steak is an easy, tasty, and affordable way to get in your daily protein. Two: the spicy Chimichurri Sauce is a win-win because it keeps really well and it's delicious not just on steak but also on chicken, fish, and veggies too. Three: tostones!

Tostones are twice-fried green plantains. If you're up for it, these are worth making and the process is easy! Seriously, impress yourself and just do the tostones. You can make them in under 20 minutes.

INGREDIENTS

2 to 3 pounds hanger steak or flank steak
1 tablespoon dried oregano
2 teaspoons cumin
2 teaspoons Kosher salt
2 tablespoons olive oil
3 tablespoons Worcestershire sauce
1 12-ounce bottle dark beer

FIXINS

Lettuce
Spinach
Radishes
Cilantro
Limes

EXTRAS

Chimichurri Sauce /165
Tostones /95
Columbian Guacamole /97

DIRECTIONS

Add all the marinade ingredients to a gallon-sized freezer bag or a large nonreactive bowl. Cover or seal and marinate for at least 2 hours.

Grill the steak on a very hot grill, 2 minutes each side.

Remove the steak to a platter.

Cover tightly with foil.

Rest for 10 minutes before slicing.

NOTES

VEGAN ADAPTABLE: Use roasted cauliflower instead of the steak. I've used purple cauliflower and it was gorgeous. Cut the cauliflower into steaks or just break it up into large pieces. Toss with salt and coconut oil. Roast for about 20 minutes at 400°F. Sprinkle with chopped parsley and serve with Chimichurri Sauce.

TOSTONES

INGREDIENTS

2 green plantains
½ cup coconut oil
Small bowl of water
Kosher salt

DIRECTIONS

Peel the green plantains and cut them into 2-inch pieces.

Heat about ½ cup of coconut oil in a cast iron or other heavy-bottomed skillet.

Set the pieces of plantain in the skillet, flat side down.

Fry them on each side until they are golden brown. (Use chopsticks or tongs to turn them.)

Remove the plantains from the oil and place them on a plate.

Use a second plate to press the fried pieces flat.

Quickly dip the smashed tostones in water and then return them to the oil.

Fry them on each side for a few minutes.

Remove the plantains and place them on a paper towel. Sprinkle with salt.

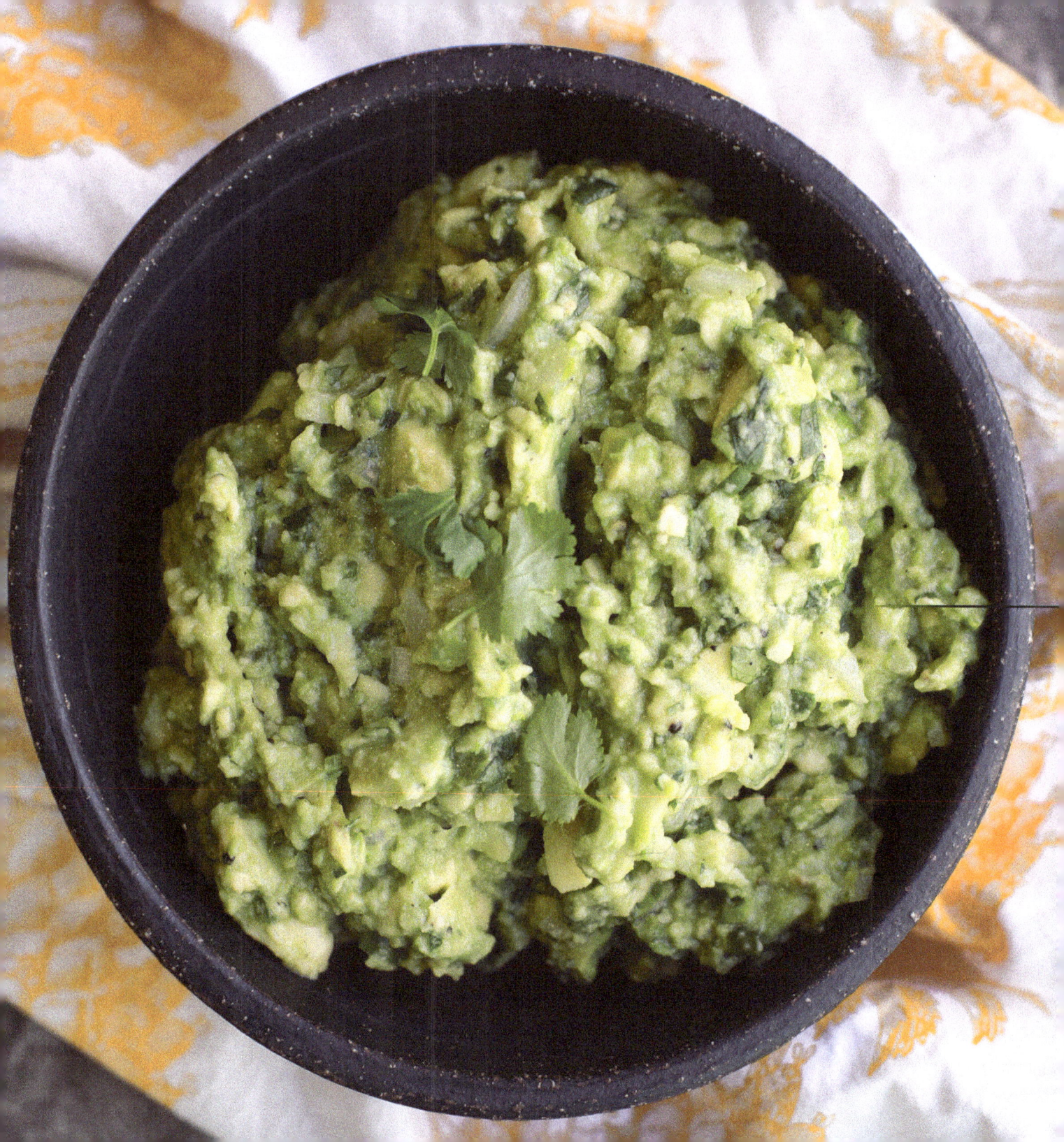

COLUMBIAN GUACAMOLE

INGREDIENTS

4 large avocados
½ Vidalia or Maui onion, finely diced
2 serrano peppers, finely diced
¼ bunch cilantro, chopped
1 lime, juiced
1 teaspoon Kosher salt

DIRECTIONS

Halve the avocados and scoop out the flesh.

Use a fork to mash the avocados until they are smooth but still a little bit chunky.

Add the onions, serrano peppers, lime, salt, and pepper. Test the salt and lime content and adjust if needed.

Add the cilantro and jalapeños and mix well.

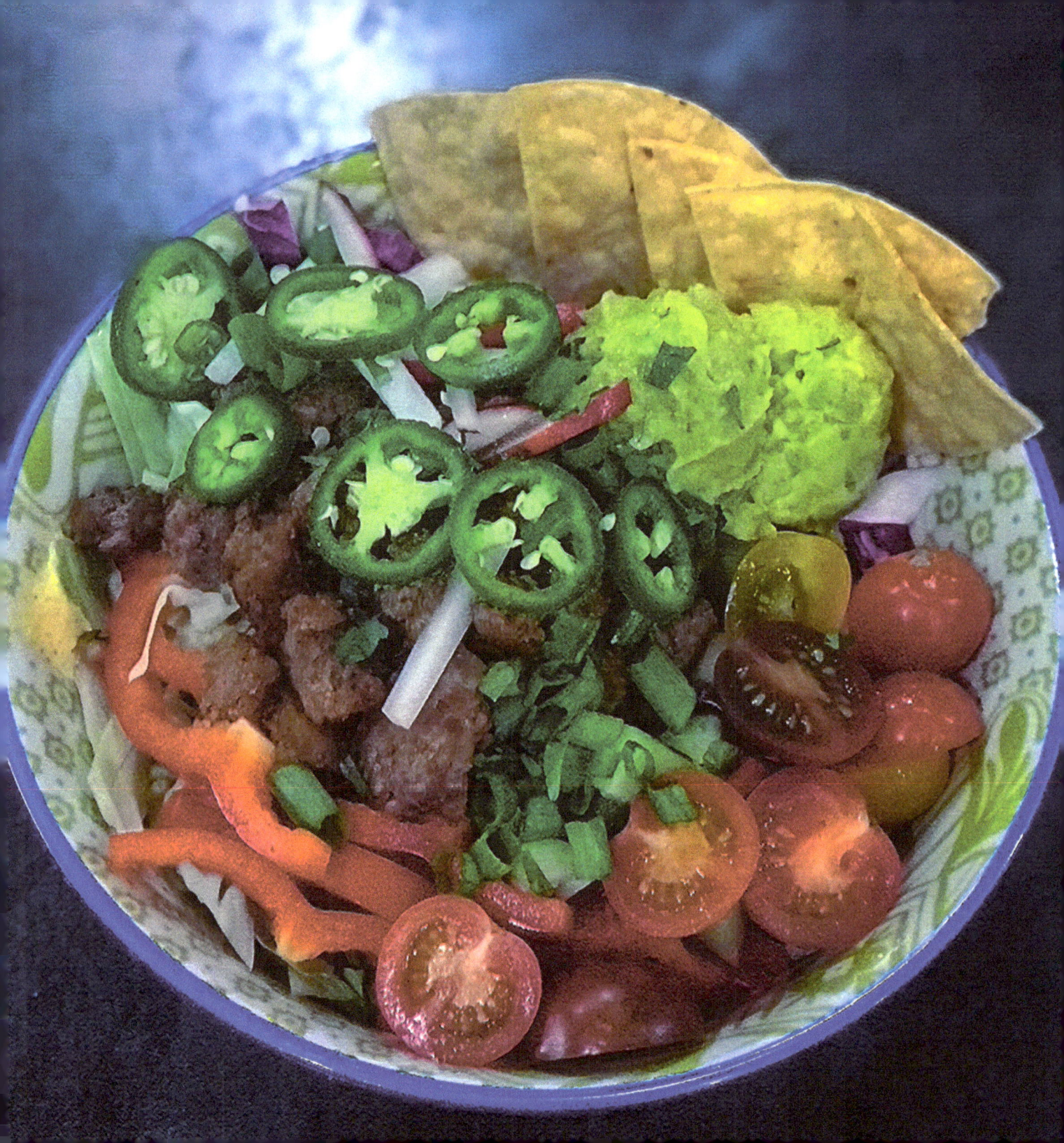

MOM-STYLE TACO

MAKES 6 TO 8 SERVINGS

This recipe takes me back to the tacos that my mom used to make when I was growing up. You know them, the ones with the crunchy shells that come in a box. I'm sure that I don't have to tell you that tacos are pretty much my most favorite food ever. I can morph literally any meal into a "taco version." It's one of my hidden talents.

This Bowl is one of my OG Beast Bowls — I was making this Beast Bowl before I even started calling them Beast Bowls!

INGREDIENTS

1 pound grass-fed ground beef or turkey
3 tablespoons salsa
1 tablespoon Taco Seasoning Mix /188

FIXINS

Romaine lettuce
Avocados
Cherry tomatoes
Red onion
Jalapeños
Grated cheddar cheese (optional)
Salsa, for dressing
Lime wedges, for garnish
Cilantro, for garnish
Green onions, for garnish

EXTRAS

Mexican Slaw /101
Mexican Guacamole /67
Avocado Cilantro Lime Crema /161
Chipotle Crema /99
Salsa Fresca /72
Roasted Corn Salsa /71

DIRECTIONS

Add the meat and taco seasoning to a heavy-bottomed skillet.

Brown on medium-high heat.

Remove from heat and stir in the salsa.

NOTES

ALTERNATIVES: You can use diced chicken or steak here as well.

VEGAN ADAPTABLE: Use ground tofu crumbles or tofu with Taco Seasoning Mix /188

MEAL PREP TIP

One of my favorite time-saving meal prep strategies is to brown up about 3 pounds of grass-fed beef. I don't do this every week, but pretty often. I usually add an onion and some salt and pepper. Then throughout the week, I can easily grab a portion out and toss it in a pan with some of my Taco Seasoning Mix or make a batch of chili when I need to whip up a quick meal.

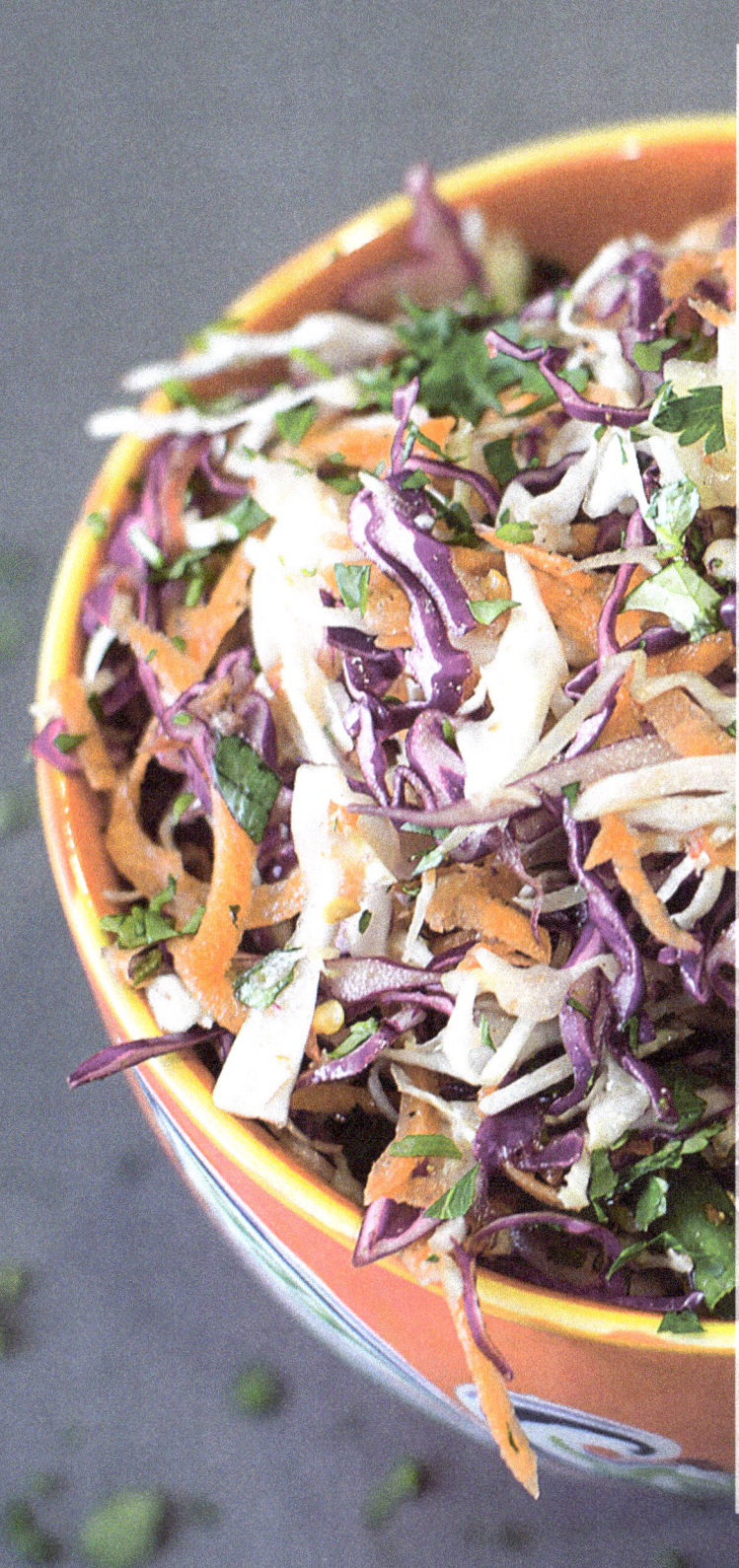

MEXICAN SLAW

INGREDIENTS

½ head red cabbage, shredded
½ head green cabbage, shredded
2 carrots, shredded
1 red pepper, julienned
1 bunch green onions, finely sliced
1 bunch cilantro, finely chopped
1 tablespoon olive oil
1 tablespoon red wine vinegar
1 lime, juiced
1 teaspoon coriander
1 teaspoon cumin
1 teaspoon Kosher salt
1 teaspoon black pepper
1 teaspoon crushed red pepper

DIRECTIONS

Add all the veggies to a large bowl.

Add the remaining ingredients and toss well with tongs.

Store all week in the refrigerator for easy servings of veggies.

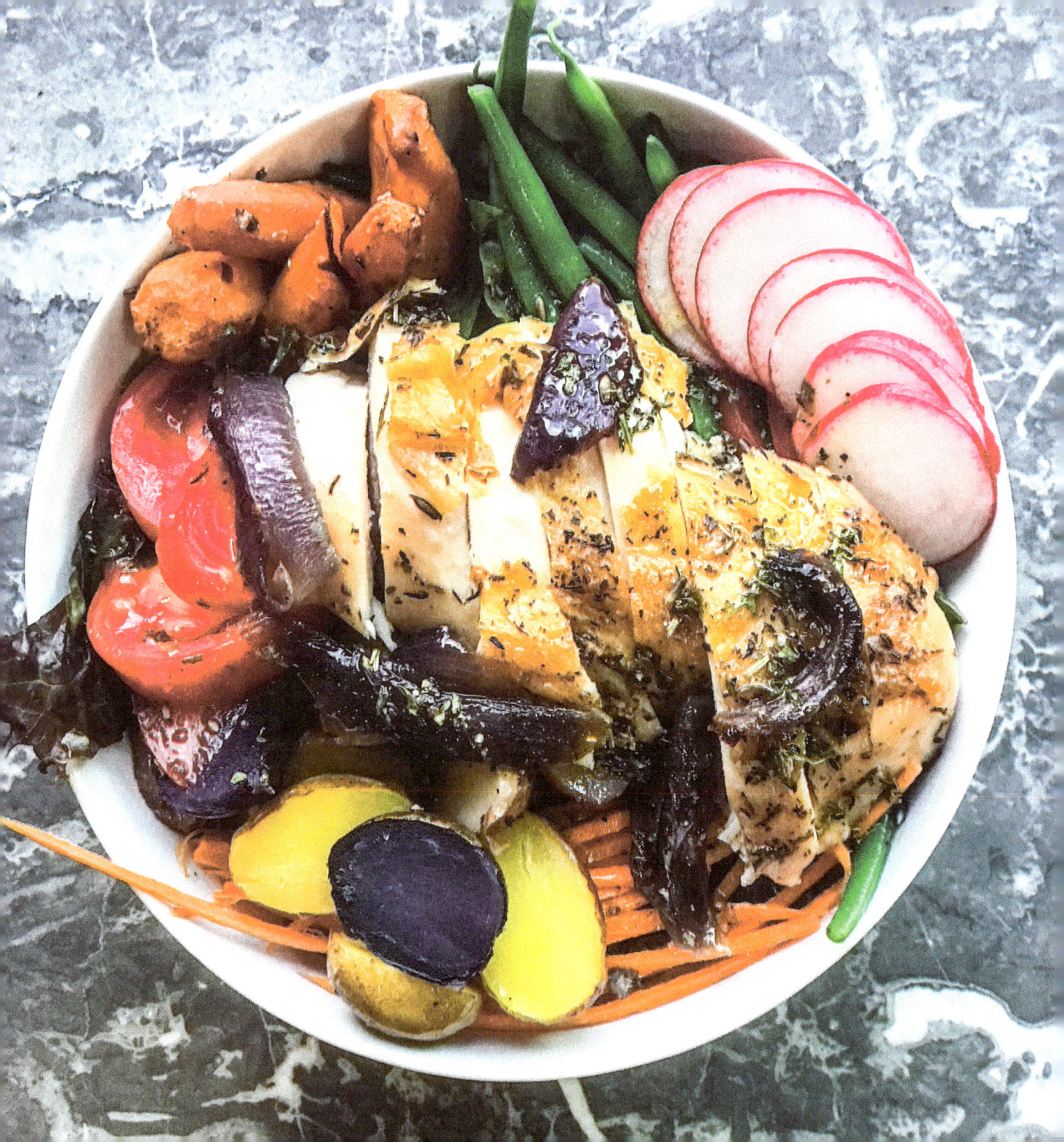

PROVENÇAL CHICKEN & VEGGIES

MAKES 6 TO 8 SERVINGS

Herbes de Provence is a classic seasoning made up of lavender, marjoram, sage, savory, and tarragon. It's easy to find in the spice aisle, or you can make your own. It tastes great on roasted chicken, fish, and vegetables. If you've never used it before, hold onto your shirt! This distinctive blend may quickly become one of your go-to seasonings.

Roasting the chicken with the bone in gives it a ton of extra flavor, but this recipe is also great with boneless, skinless chicken breasts or thighs.

INGREDIENTS

8 chicken breasts, bone in, skin on
2 cups baby potatoes, halved
1 red onion, sliced or diced into bite-sized pieces
2 cups carrots, peeled and cut on the diagonal
2 tablespoons coconut oil
½ tablespoon Kosher salt
4 tablespoons Herbes de Provence /185

FIXINS

Shredded carrots
Tomatoes
Radishes
Red peppers
Roasted potatoes
Roasted carrots
Roasted onions

EXTRAS

Herbes de Provence Vinaigrette /144
Blanched Green Beans /105

DIRECTIONS

Preheat the oven to 425°F.

Prepare the vegetables and season them lightly with salt, pepper, Herbes de Provence, and a little bit of coconut oil. Toss and place on a sheet pan.

Sprinkle the chicken with Herbes de Provence, salt, and a little oil.

Place the chicken on a rack above the vegetables.

Place the pan in the oven and roast for about 25 to 40 minutes (depending on the oven). The chicken should have an internal temperature of 165°F.

Remove the chicken and let it rest 10 minutes before removing it from the bone.

NOTES

PRO TIPS: A meat thermometer is essential here if you want perfect chicken.

Line the pan with parchment paper for easier cleanup.

ROASTING 101

OPTION 1: Place the vegetables on a sheet pan, then place a bakery cooling rack over the top. Position the chicken on the rack. This allows the juice and flavors from the chicken to drip onto the vegetables during roasting and gives everything a nice flavor.

OPTION 2: Place the chicken and veggies on separate sheet pans. I do this a lot because I'm the mom of a vegan. I still like to elevate my chicken above the sheet pan with a cooling rack, because this allows the skin to get crispier. YUM! If you're using separate pans, the veggies should be done after about 20 minutes.

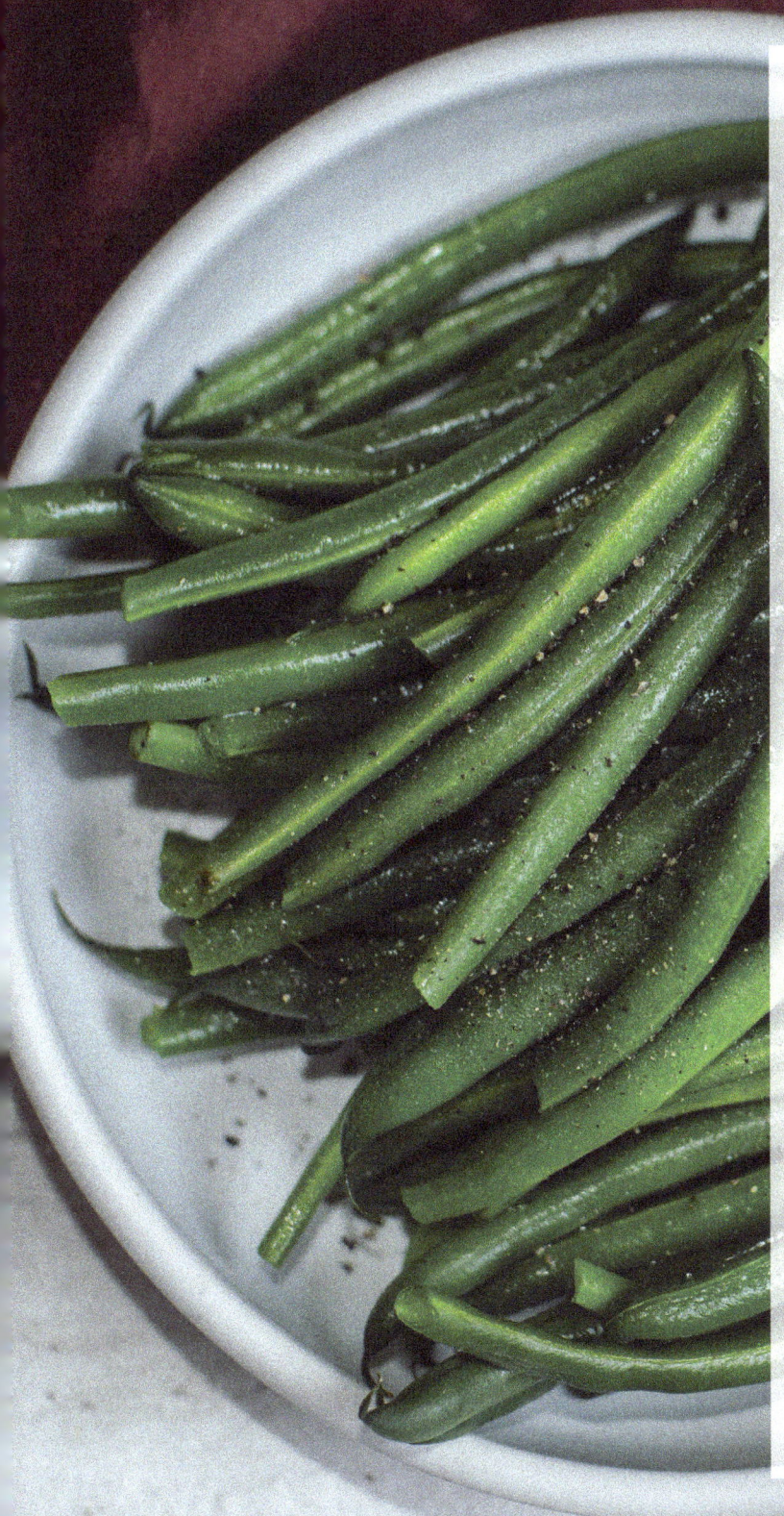

BLANCHED GREEN BEANS

INGREDIENTS

2 pounds green beans or French haricots verts
2 tablespoons of Kosher salt
Large bowl of ice water

DIRECTIONS

Add 2 large tablespoons of salt to 6 cups of water and bring it to a boil.

Get a large bowl of ice water ready and set it aside.

Once the water is boiling, add the green beans and boil them for about 4 minutes.

Remove the green beans from the water using tongs or a large slotted spoon. Place them immediately into the ice water.

Remove them from the ice water and serve.

BLANCHING is a method of cooking vegetables briefly in salted, boiling water and then plunging them quickly into ice water. This method retains the beautiful bright color of the vegetable and works great on beans, broccoli, and bok choy cabbage.

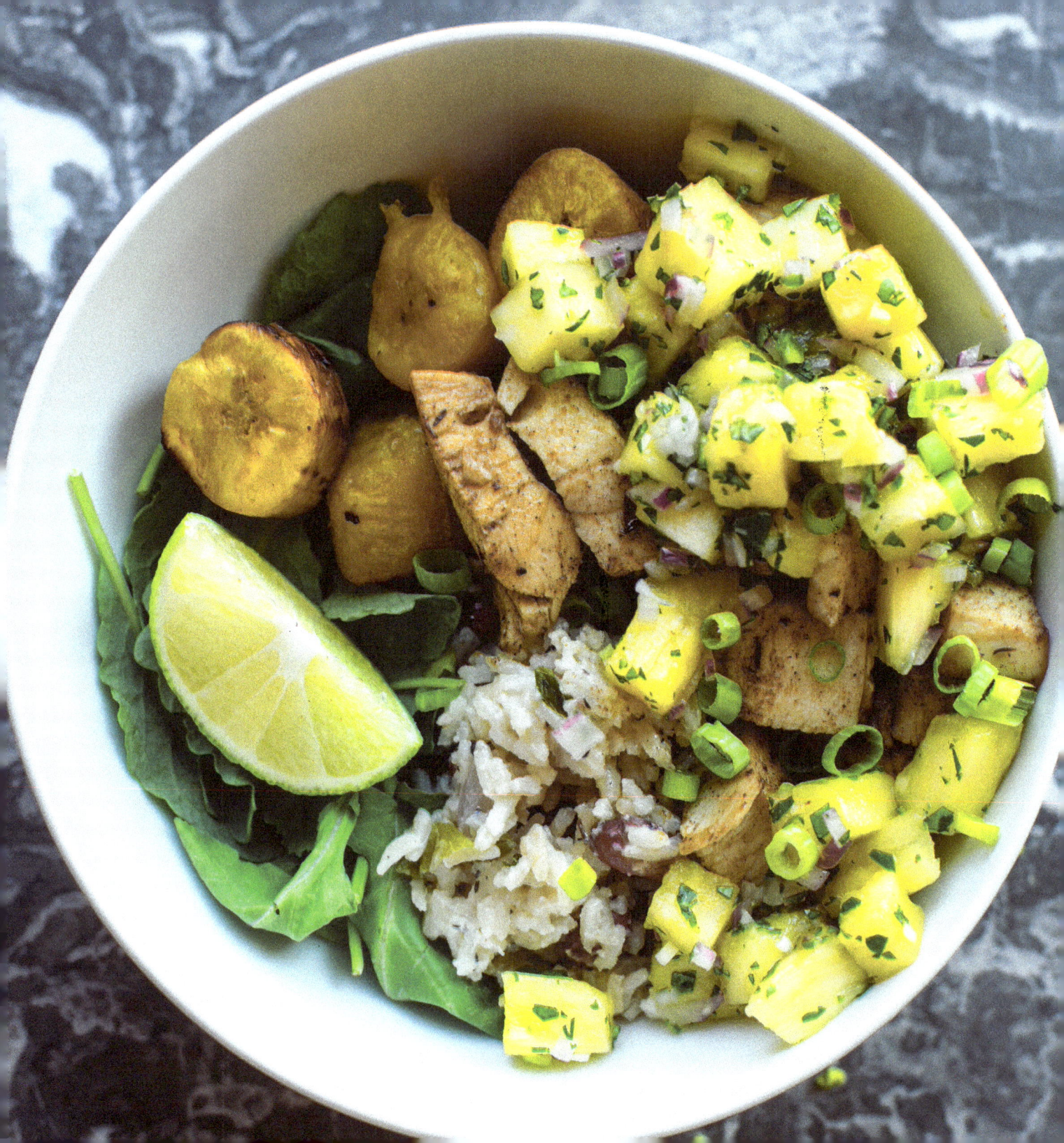

JAMAICAN JERK CHICKEN

MAKES 6 TO 8 SERVINGS

This spicy jerk chicken is served with Roasted Plantains and Jamaican Rice & Peas and then topped with a spicy-sweet Pineapple Salsa, creating a bowl full of island flavor. A squeeze of lime really brings all the flavors together.

Don't let the carbs in this one scare you off, make them work for you! Just eat this Bowl before hitting the gym! If it's still too many carbs for you, cut down on the rice. Notice I didn't say "leave out the plantains," because plantains rock!

INGREDIENTS

1 whole chicken, whole or cut up
2 teaspoons coconut oil
2 tablespoons Jamaican Jerk Seasoning Mix /187

FIXINS

Baby kale greens
Romaine lettuce
Spinach
Shredded carrots
Red bell pepper
Red cabbage

EXTRAS

Roasted Plantains /109
Pineapple Salsa /110
Jamaican Rice and Peas /113

DIRECTIONS

Preheat the oven to 425°F.

Prepare a pan for roasting.

GET READY TO ROAST: Place a cooling rack over a sheet pan that has been lined with parchment paper, or use a roasting pan fitted with a roasting rack.

Rub the chicken with Jamaican Jerk Seasoning Mix.

Place the chicken on the roasting pan.

Roast until the temperature at the thigh of the chicken is 165°F.

NOTES

USE A THERMOMETER: The cooking time will vary depending on whether or not you are roasting a whole bird or roasting cut up pieces. When the chicken reaches the proper cooking temperature (165°F at the thickest part of the thigh), remove it from the oven. Let it rest at least 10 minutes before slicing. Slice and store any extra chicken for use in meals the rest of the week.

SPATCHCOCK IT: This is a process where the backbone is removed and the chicken is laid flat during the roasting. It cuts the cooking time almost in half and makes it easier to cook the chicken evenly on the grill.

PRO TIP: Have the butcher cut up your chicken for you.

SHORTCUT: Buy a pre-made jerk seasoning.

ALTERNATIVE: Use diced chicken breasts or thighs and pan sauté them to save time. This seasoning mix is also amazing on a batch of chicken wings.

VEGAN ADAPTABLE: Use sliced portobello mushrooms instead of the chicken.

ROASTED PLANTAINS

INGREDIENTS

4 ripe plantains
2 teaspoons coconut oil
1 teaspoon Kosher salt

DIRECTIONS

Preheat the oven to 425°F.

Peel the plantains and cut them into 2-inch pieces.

Toss them in coconut oil and salt.

Roast the plantains in a cast iron skillet or on a baking sheet for about 20 minutes. Toss about halfway through cooking. Oven temperatures vary, so watch carefully.

NOTES

PRO TIP: These can be cooked in the oven right alongside the chicken. Just make sure you keep an eye on them and take them out when they are golden brown.

PINEAPPLE SALSA

INGREDIENTS

2 cups fresh pineapple, diced
2 serrano peppers, finely diced
⅓ cup red onion, finely diced
2 tablespoons cilantro, minced
1 lime, juiced
2 teaspoons coconut oil
1 teaspoon Kosher salt
¼ teaspoon black pepper

DIRECTIONS

Dice and chop all the fruits and vegetables.

Toss in a large nonreactive bowl.

Add lime juice, coconut oil, salt, and pepper to taste. Toss.

Store any leftovers in an airtight container in the refrigerator.

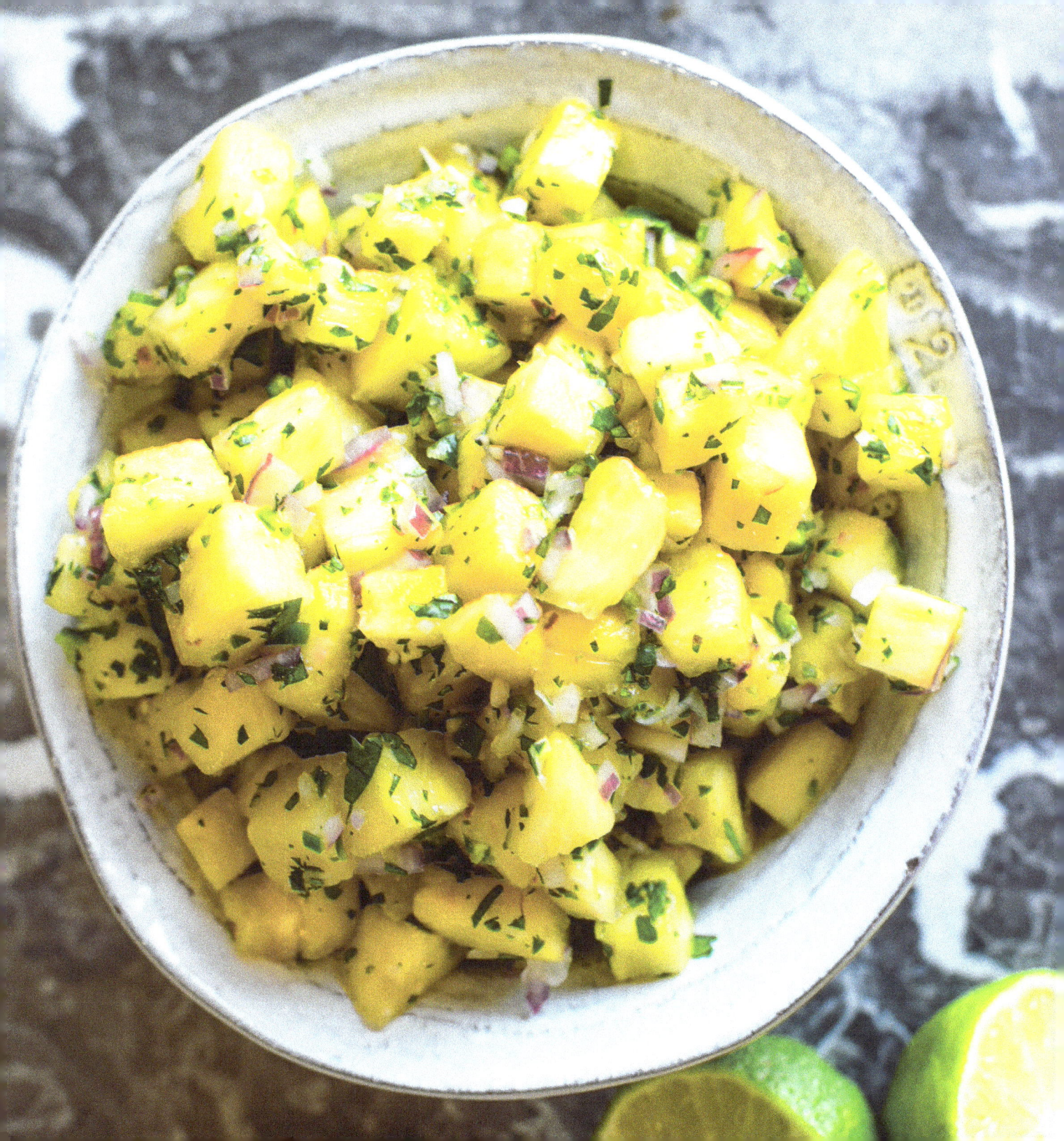

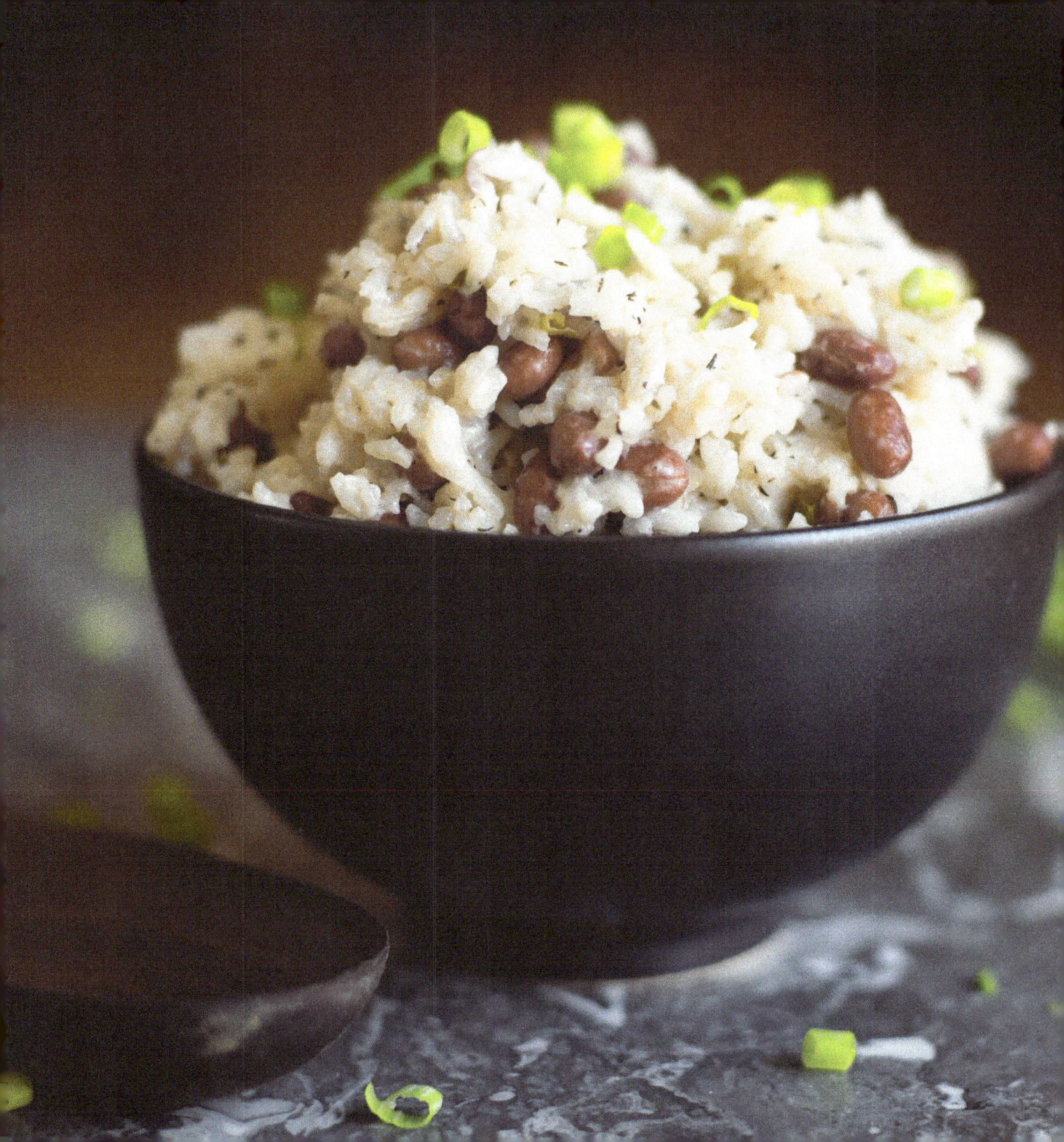

JAMAICAN RICE & PEAS

INGREDIENTS

1 14-ounce can small red beans
1 14-ounce can coconut milk
Water, enough to bring liquid to 4 cups
1 tablespoon coconut oil
½ small yellow onion, diced
2 cloves garlic, pressed
2 cups long grain white rice
2 green onions, sliced
1 teaspoon dried thyme
1 teaspoon Kosher salt

DIRECTIONS

Drain the red beans, reserving the liquid into a 4-cup measuring cup. Set the beans aside.

Combine the liquid from the red beans and the coconut milk in a large measuring cup.

Add enough water to the measuring cup to bring the liquid up to 4 total cups. Set aside.

Add the coconut oil to a medium-sized saucepan and heat it on medium-high.

Add the yellow onion and garlic and cook them for a few minutes until they are fragrant and translucent.

Add the rice and cook it for a few minutes until the rice is coated with oil and slightly toasted.

Add the beans, green onions, thyme, salt, and liquid to the pan. Stir.

Bring to a boil.

Reduce the heat to simmer, cover, and cook until all liquid is absorbed, about 20 minutes. Stir occasionally.

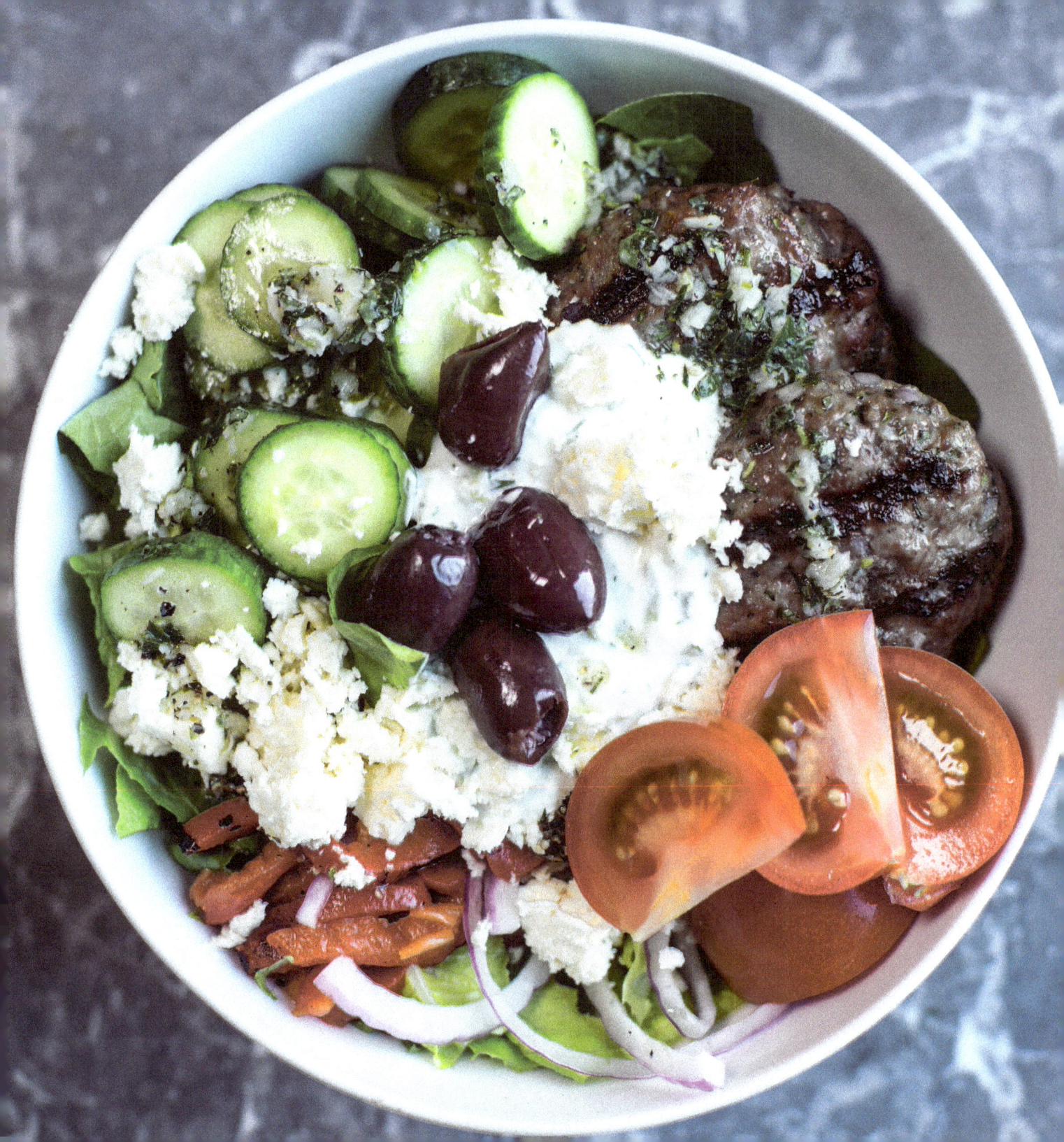

GREEK LAMB BURGER

MAKES 6 TO 8 SERVINGS

This Bowl has all the goodness of a gyro but without the carb coma. The Greek Vinaigrette, Tzatziki, feta cheese, and Kalamata olives are all major flavor bombs. You can also add some couscous if you're looking for a little more carbs here.

If you've been afraid to try lamb, this is your chance to change your mind. Because the meat is seasoned with strong flavors like garlic, oregano, and lemon, you end up with a very balanced flavor. Paired with the creamy Tzatziki and salty feta — you really can't go wrong.

INGREDIENTS

1 to 1½ pounds grass-fed ground beef
1 to 1½ pounds pasture raised ground lamb
1 tablespoon dried oregano
2 teaspoons Kosher salt
2 teaspoons crushed red pepper
½ red onion, finely diced
4 cloves garlic, minced
1 tablespoon lemon zest

FIXINS

Cucumbers
Couscous
Feta cheese
Kalamata olives
Lettuce or mixed greens
Red onion
Roasted red pepper
Tomatoes
Pita (optional)

EXTRAS

Tzatziki /169
Greek Vinaigrette /144

DIRECTIONS

Add the meat and all the spices to a large bowl.

Add the onions, garlic, and lemon zest to the meat. Mix well.

Use your hands or a large cookie scoop to form the meat mixture into patties.

Grill, bake, or pan-fry. My favorite is grilling!

Adjust the timing as needed.

NOTES

IN THE OVEN: 425°F for about 20 minutes.

STOVE TOP: Medium-high heat for about 2 minutes each side.

GRILL: High heat for about 2 minutes each side. Lower the heat if you are using ground chicken. Cook the chicken for 3 to 4 minutes on each side.

ALTERNATIVE: These patties are also delicious when made with either all ground beef or ground chicken. You can also use whole chicken thighs or chicken tenderloins. If you're using pieces of chicken, add a few teaspoons of oil to the seasoning, toss to coat and then bake the chicken in the oven.

VEGAN ADAPTABLE: Season diced eggplant, red bell peppers, and red onions with the seasonings. Roast at 400°F for about 20 minutes.

MEET MEAT

Have you ever walked right past the butcher's counter because it felt too intimidating? If you've ever been confused about how to pick meat, I can help you. This meat primer covers a few of my go-to meat choices – I buy these over and over again because they are easy to cook, even if you are a beginner.

Download my comprehensive meat buying guide from the blog and never let your protein go to waste again! Get it at FoodologyGeek.com/BBN

PRO TIP: All meat should be at room temp before cooking.

GROUND

Think meatballs, meatloaf, or neatly portioned patties that can be grilled, baked, or cooked on the stove-top.

Ground beef is versatile and cooks really quickly. Beef cuts vary in leaness. I typically buy a 90:10 or an 85:15 ratio of Protein:Fat.

Chicken, turkey, lamb, and pork can also be purchased ground.

STEAK CUTS

My favorite beef steaks:

Chateaubriand
Filet
London broil
Flat Iron AKA hanger steak

A few great pork steaks:

Pork loin
Bone-in pork chops

ROASTS

Roast cuts are perfect for the slow cooker or Instant pot:

Beef or pork shoulder
Brisket
Tri-tip
Pork tenderloin

POULTRY

The most common cuts that I keep in the freezer:

Whole roasting chicken
Cut up fryer chicken
Bone-in breasts and thighs
Boneless breasts and thighs
Frozen chicken breasts and tenders

SEAFOOD

Frozen fish and other seafood is a massive time saver:

Frozen salmon
Frozen halibut
Frozen cod
Frozen uncooked shrimp

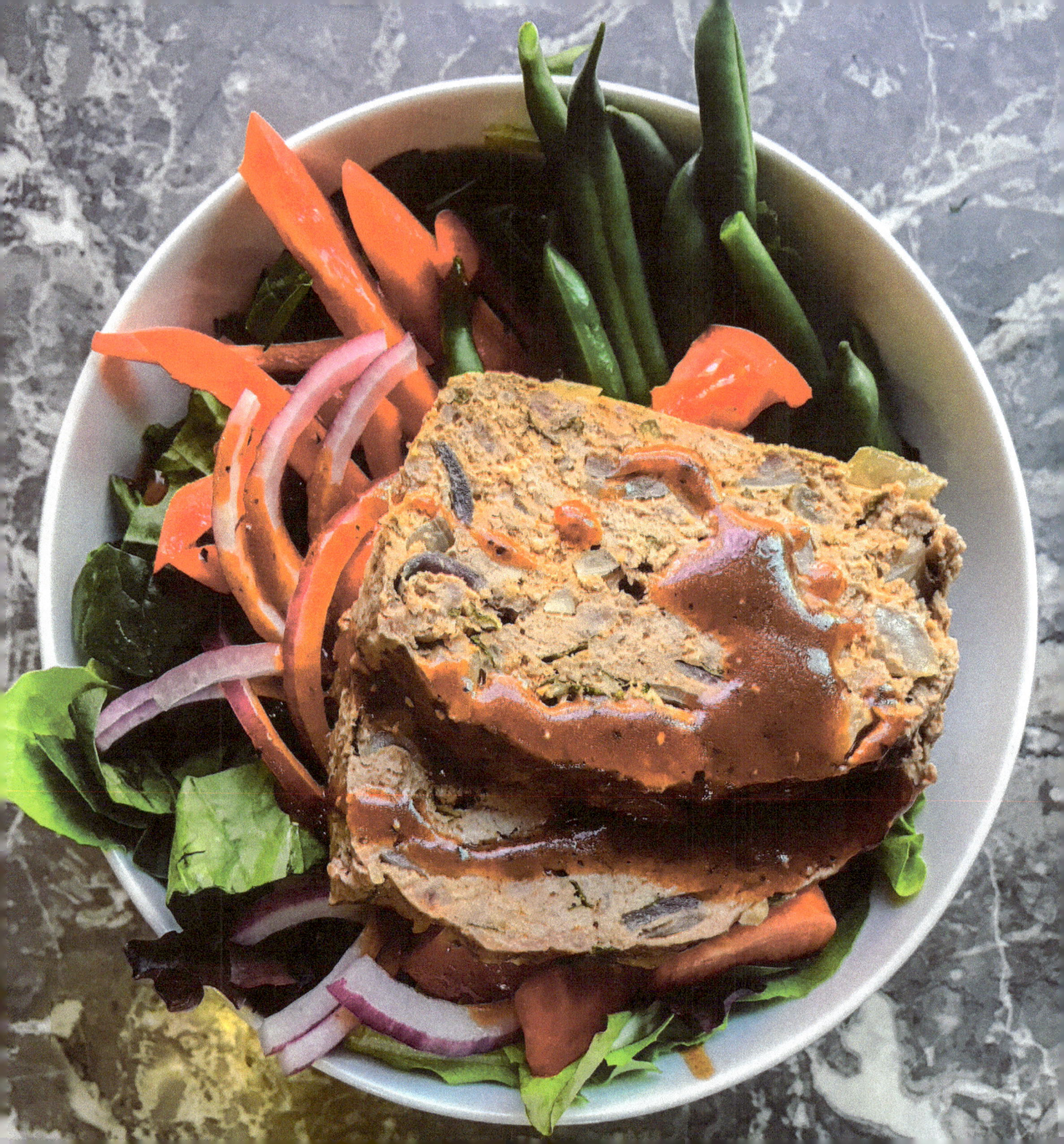

PALEO MEATLOAF

MAKES 6 TO 8 SERVINGS

This recipe takes me back to being a kid of the 80s. I can still remember riding around the neighborhood on my green bike with the glittery banana seat and the ape hanger handlebars. Can you relate? My brother and I had to be home when the street lights came on, and we were always starving.

Meatloaf was a staple in my family's weekly dinner rotation. Some dishes are iconic for an era. Meat in the form of a loaf definitely fits right in with the 80s genre. The thing I remember most is that no two meatloaves were ever alike. But this one is delicious!

INGREDIENTS

3 pounds ground beef
⅓ cup almond flour
2 eggs, lightly beaten
1 onion, finely chopped
3 cloves garlic, minced
⅔ cup fresh parsley, chopped
2 tablespoons Worcestershire sauce
1 tablespoon chili powder
1 teaspoon paprika
1 tablespoon Kosher salt
1 teaspoon crushed red pepper

FIXINS

Romaine lettuce
Spinach
Red onion
Tomatoes
Red peppers

EXTRAS

Spicy Tomato Jam /179
Tomato Balsamic Viniagrette /147
Onion Jam /177
Blanched Green Beans /105

DIRECTIONS

Preheat oven to 350°F.

In a large bowl, mix together the remaining ingredients for the meatloaf. I usually use my hands.

Divide the mixture in half and place it in two loaf pans. Place the pans on a large baking sheet.

Bake for 1 hour.

Remove from the oven and drain off any excess fat.

Let the meatloaf rest for about 30 minutes before slicing.

NOTES

ALTERNATIVES: You can eat this meatloaf with a heaping side of green beans and mashed potatoes or try the Cauliflower Smash /121.

I must confess that I love a good meatloaf sandwich! Just grab some toasted sourdough and slather it with onion jam and a few ripe tomatoes. Yum!

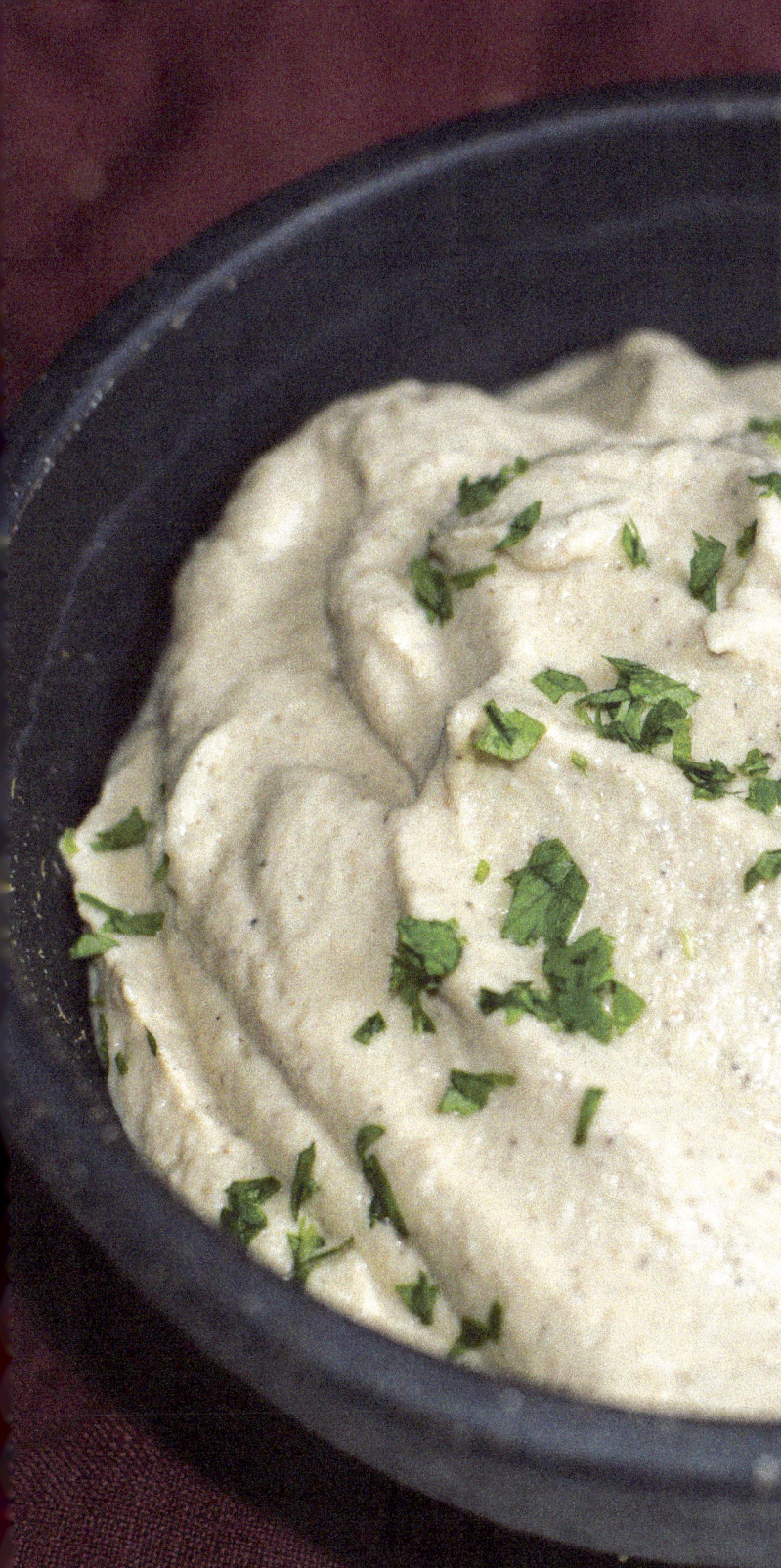

CAULIFLOWER SMASH

INGREDIENTS

2 heads of cauliflower, removed from the core
2 teaspoons of avocado oil
2 teaspoons of salt
2 to 4 teaspoons of butter
½ cup of heavy cream

DIRECTIONS

Preheat the oven to 450F

Add the cauliflower florets to a large roasting pan or a baking sheet.

Toss with the avocado oil and a little salt and pepper.

Roast for 20 minutes, until the cauliflower is a light golden brown.

Add the roasted cauliflower florets to the work bowl of a food processor or high powered blender.

Add the butter and heavy cream.

Process until the cauliflower is smooth and creamy.

NON DAIRY OPTIONS: Coconut milk or any non-dairy milk can be used to replace the butter and the heavy cream.

ROASTED GARLIC VERSION: Wrap 4 to 6 whole garlic cloves and a little oil in a foil. Add this packet and roast with the cauliflower. Toss the soft roasted garlic into the food processor with the cauliflower.

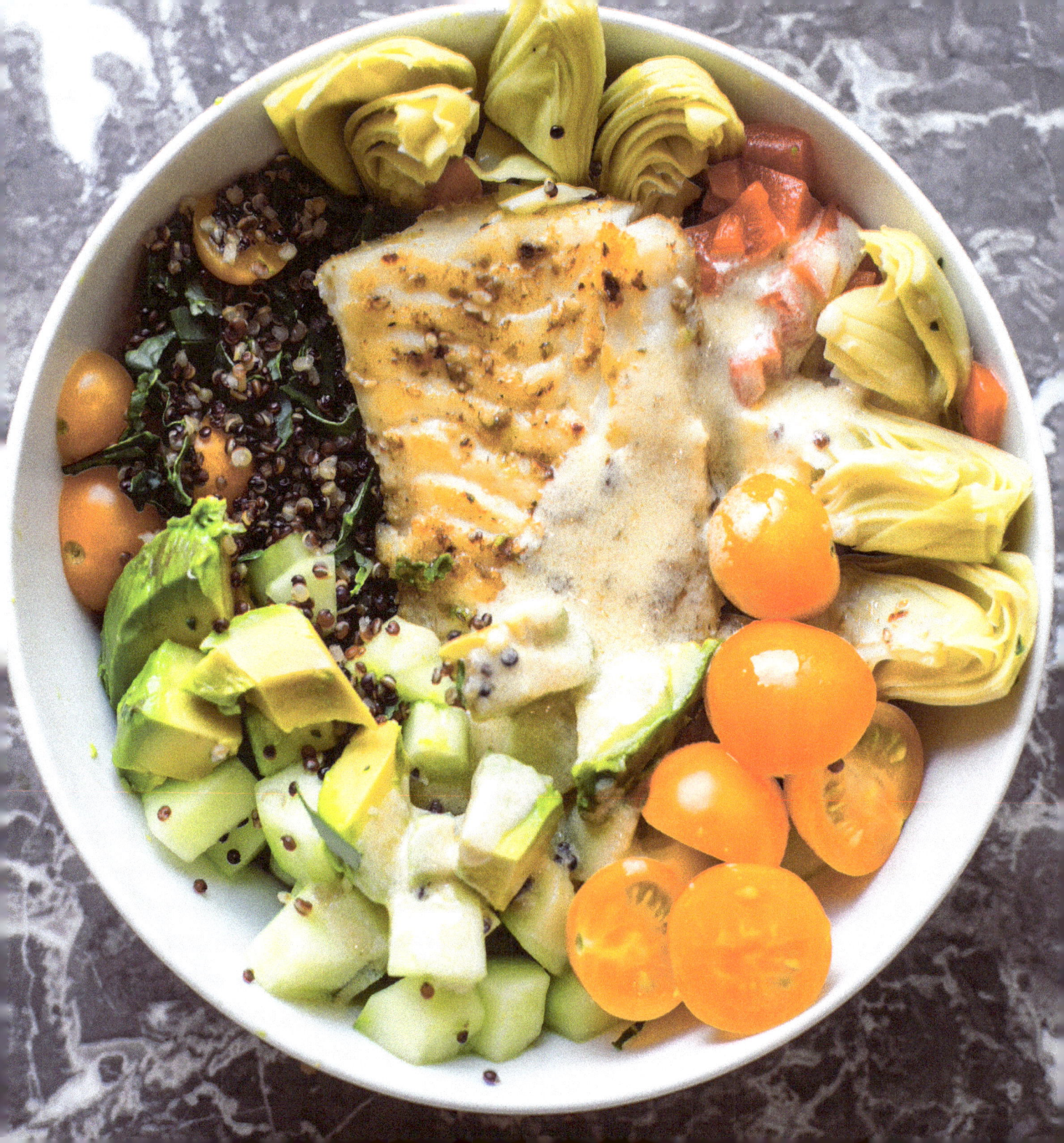

MEDITERRANEAN FISH

MAKES 6 TO 8 SERVINGS

Using seasoning mixes in meal prep is a real game-changer, making it so easy to add a ton of flavor to what would otherwise be just a boring protein.

The Mediterranean Seasoning Mix is what makes this Beast Bowl spectacular! This Bowl is full of healthy fats and tons of veggies on a bed of quinoa, and the Lemon Tahini Dressing is great on so many things. This dressing is a staple in our house, where we also use it on grilled chicken and roasted veggies.

INGREDIENTS

- 2 to 3 teaspoons of avocado oil
- 2 to 3 pounds white fish, such as mahi-mahi, cod, or halibut
- 2 to 3 teaspoons Mediterranean Seasoning Mix /185

FIXINS

- Quinoa, cooked
- Lacinato kale
- Cucumbers
- Cherry tomatoes
- Avocado
- Artichoke hearts, quartered (canned or frozen)
- Roasted red peppers

EXTRAS

Lemon Tahini Dressing /171

DIRECTIONS

Sprinkle the fish generously with Mediterranean Seasoning Mix.

Cook the fish in a sauté pan or in the oven.

NOTES

STOVE TOP: Heat a few tablespoons of avocado oil or butter in a medium sauté pan. Add the fish and cook for 3 minutes on each side. Rest for 5 minutes before serving.

OVEN: Preheat the oven to 425°F. Bake the fish for 10 minutes on a parchment-lined baking sheet.

ALTERNATIVE: Use chicken, shrimp or tofu.

PRO TIP: You are going to want to make extra of this seasoning mix and have it around all the time. Just go ahead and double it! It is so good on roasted Yukon Gold potatoes with a side of either Buffalo or Paleo Ranch. Snack heaven!

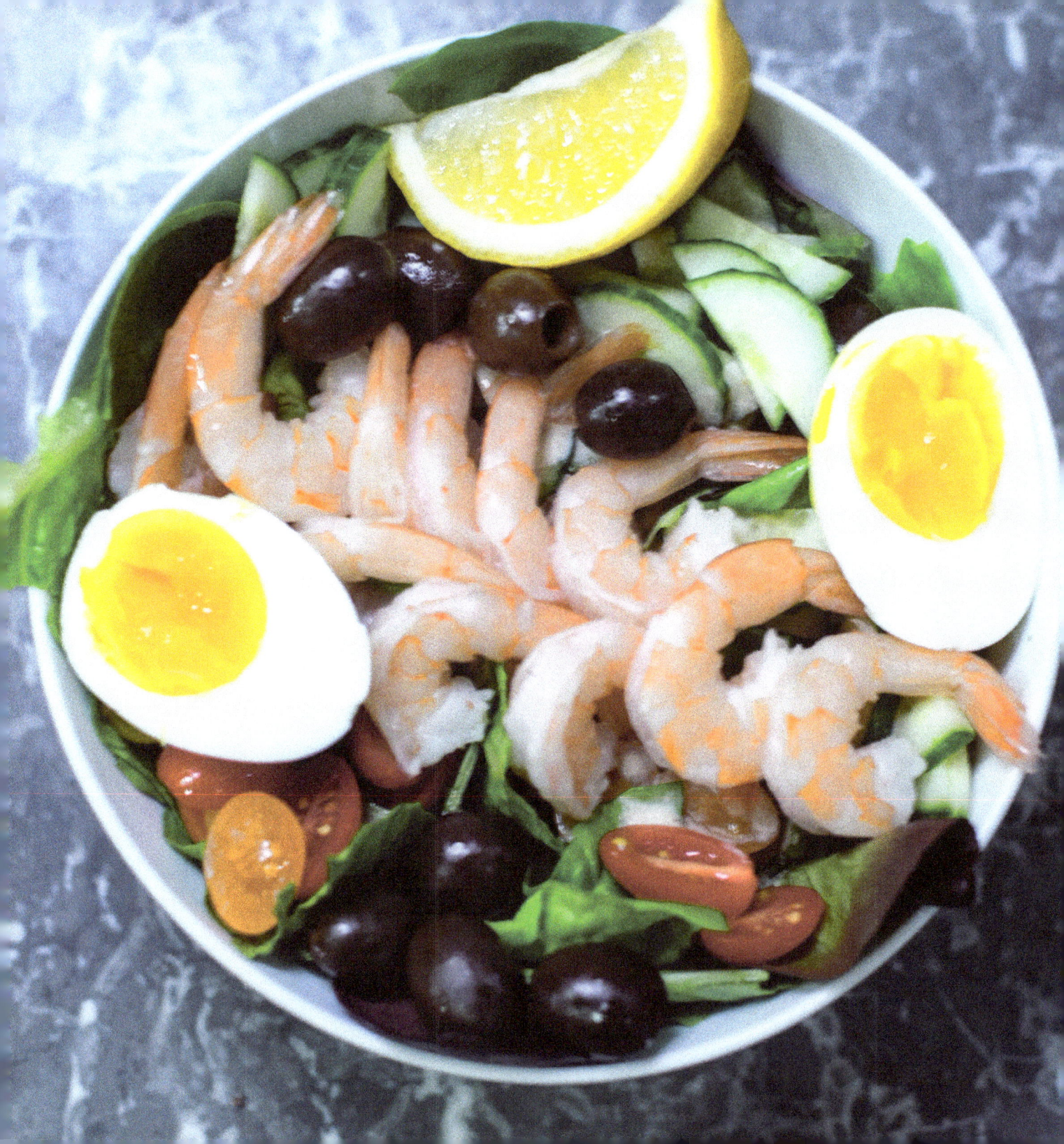

SHRIMP LOUIE

MAKES 6 TO 8 SERVINGS

Always pronounced with a pretentious "loo-ee!" I love the fresh seafood and zesty lemon paired with the uncomplicated Louie Dressing. I can almost smell the saltwater right now! This Beast Bowl is super simple to put together, and if you buy frozen cooked shrimp, you just defrost them, give them a quick rinse, and toss them in the bowl.

INGREDIENTS

- 2 to 3 pounds shrimp, tail on, cleaned, cooked and chilled
- 4 to 8 hard boiled eggs, halved

FIXINS

- Romaine lettuce
- Avocados
- Cherry tomatoes
- Black olives
- Lemon wedges

LOUIE DRESSING

- 1 cup mayonnaise
- ¼ cup chili sauce
- ½ lemon, juiced

Whisk all the ingredients together.

DIRECTIONS

Use frozen, cooked, and already cleaned shrimp.

Thaw, rinse, and drain the shrimp.

Squeeze a few tablespoons of lemon juice over the chilled shrimp and toss to coat.

NOTES

SHORTCUT: Buy frozen shrimp, then just thaw and rinse.

PRO TIPS: Thawing shrimp is quick and easy. Place the shrimp in a large plastic bag and then dunk the whole thing in a bowl of room temperature water. You can come back in about 20 to 30 minutes, and they will be all thawed and ready to go.

For perfect soft boiled eggs that peel easily, bring the water to a boil before adding eggs. Add the eggs and boil them for 7 to 8 minutes. 7 minutes gives you a softer, runnier yolk.

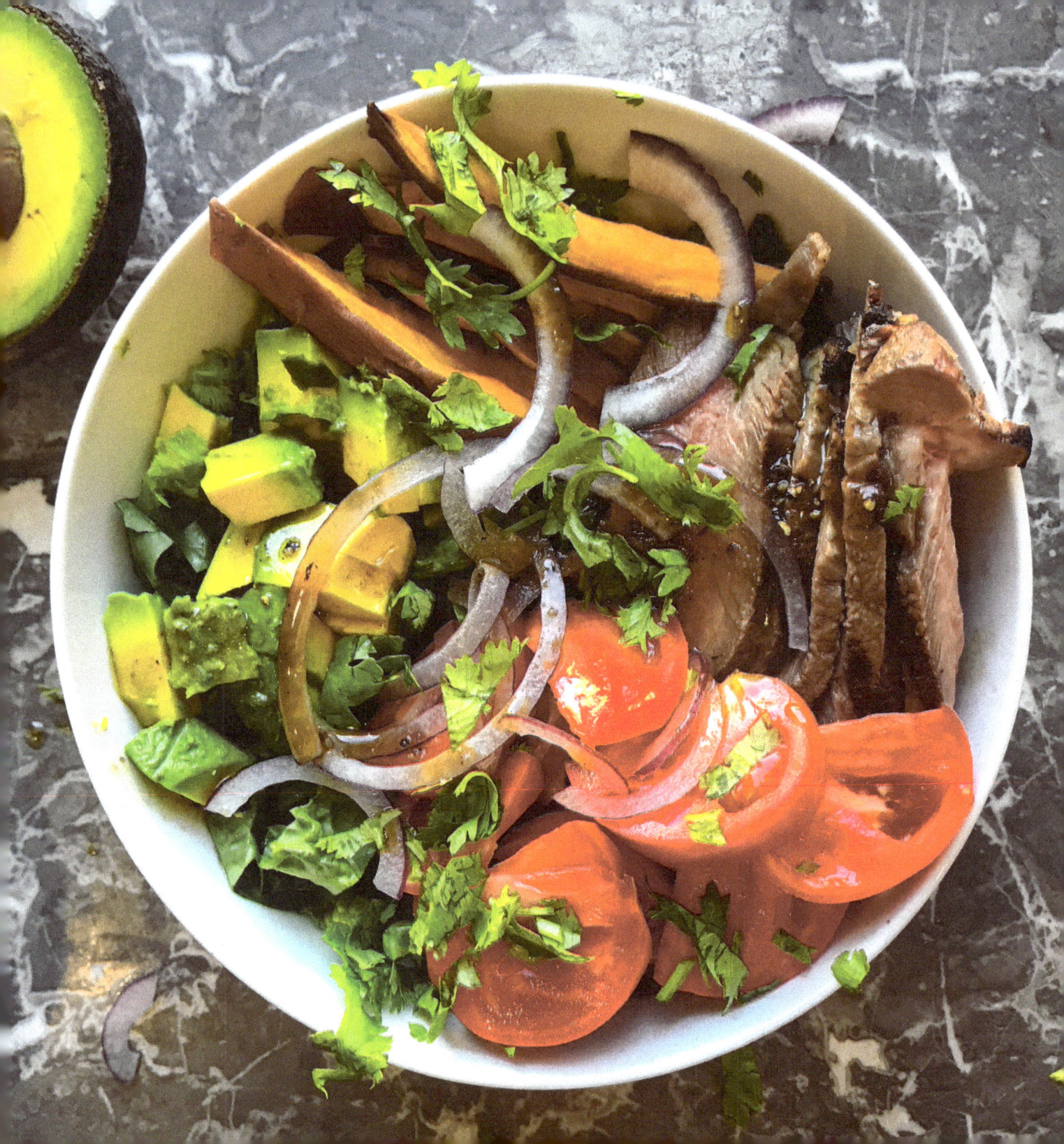

STEAK & SWEET POTATO

MAKES 6 TO 8 SERVINGS

Steak is probably my favorite protein! For this recipe, you can use any cut of steak that you like and know how to cook well. For this Bowl, I chose a Chateaubriand cut — it's flavorful and tender, plus easy to cook.

Sweet Potato Fries provide the perfect complement to the steak in this Beast Bowl. Add the tangy Balsamic Vinaigrette and a dose of fresh healthy vegetables, and you just might have the best Beast Bowl in this book. The flavor combination can't be beaten!

INGREDIENTS

- 2 pounds Chateaubriand steak OR any other variety that you like.
- ¼ cup balsamic vinegar
- 2 teaspoons coconut oil
- 2 teaspoons mushroom salt or plain Kosher salt
- 1 teaspoon black pepper

VEGAN ADAPTABLE: Sauté mushrooms instead of using steak.

DIRECTIONS

Rub the steak with mushroom salt and pepper.

Place it in a gallon-sized freezer bag or a large nonreactive bowl.

Add the balsamic vinegar, coconut oil, salt, and pepper.

Toss to coat and let it marinate for about 2 hours.

PRO TIP: *Steak should be at room temperature for at least an hour before you grill it.*

Grill on high heat. For medium-rare steaks, cook to an internal temperature of 135°F.

Tender Cuts - 4 ounces		Tough Cuts - 4 ounces	
Sirloin Tip	9g Fat / 23g Protein	Bottom Round	14g Fat / 23g Protein
Top Round	9g Fat / 25g Protein	Top Sirloin	15g Fat / 24g Protein
Filet Mignon	21g Fat / 22g Protein	NY Strip	5g Fat / 21g Protein
Hanger	14g Fat / 39g Protein	Skirt	9g Fat / 24g Protein

BEAST BOWL NUTRITION | CHAPTER 4 | CORE PROTEINS & EXTRAS

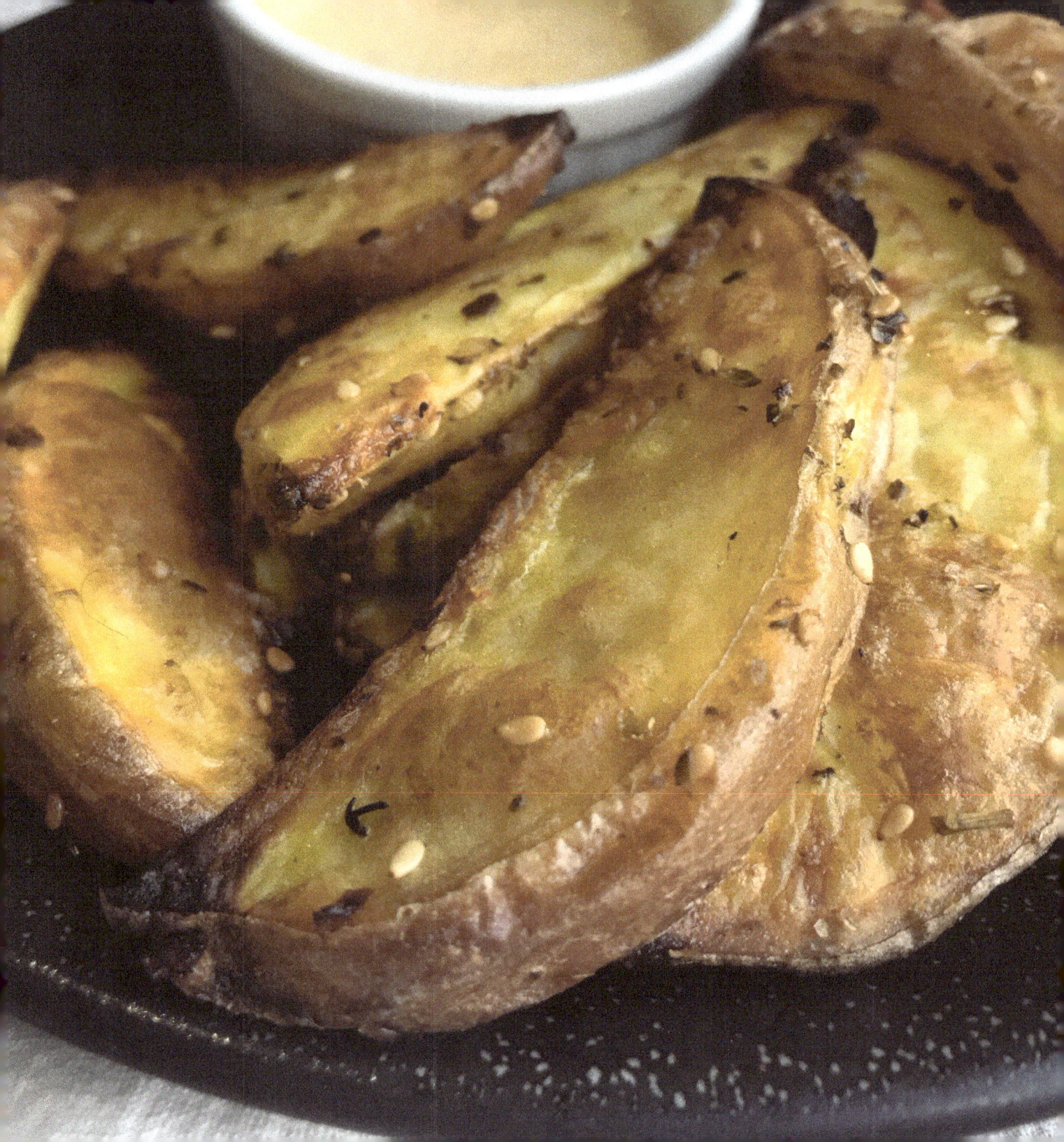

OVEN ROASTED POTATOES

INGREDIENTS

4-6 small Yukon Gold potatoes
2 teaspoons coconut oil or avocado oil
1 teaspoon Kosher salt

DIRECTIONS

Preheat the oven to 425°F.

Wash and dry the potatoes.

Cut the potatoes into fries or cubes.

Place the cut potatoes on a parchment-lined baking sheet.

Drizzle them with the oil, sprinkle with salt, and toss to coat.

Spread the potatoes evenly on the baking sheet.

Roast for about 15 to 20 minutes until they are tender and golden brown.

NOTES

ALTERNATIVE: Use the Mediterranean Seasoning /185 OR the Barbecue Seasoning /187 instead of salt.

SERVING SUGGESTION: Serve with one of the mayo-based sauces like Buffalo Ranch /156 or Paleo Ranch /155.

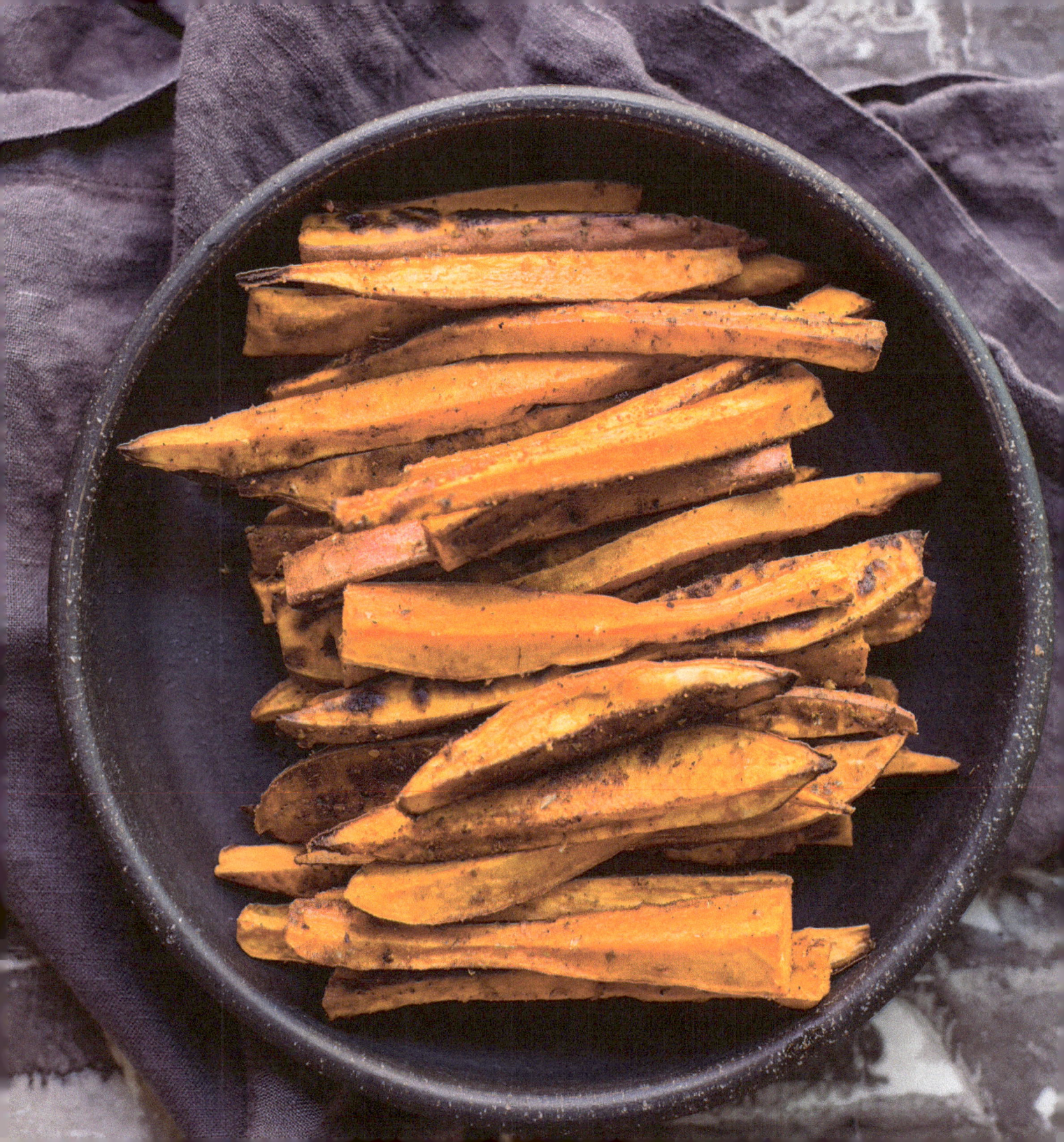

SWEET POTATO FRIES

INGREDIENTS

2 small sweet potatoes
2 teaspoons coconut oil or avocado oil
1 teaspoon Kosher salt

DIRECTIONS

Preheat the oven to 425°F.

Wash and dry the sweet potatoes.

Cut the sweet potatoes into fries.

Place the fries on a parchment-lined baking sheet.

Drizzle them with coconut oil, sprinkle with salt, and toss to coat.

Spread the fries evenly on the baking sheet.

Roast for about 15 to 20 minutes until they are tender and golden brown.

NOTES

PRO TIP: Cut the sweet potatoes into cubes to make a batch of roasted sweet potatoes.

SHORTCUT: Use frozen sweet potato fries.

ALTERNATIVE: Use the Barbecue Spice Rub /187 instead of salt.

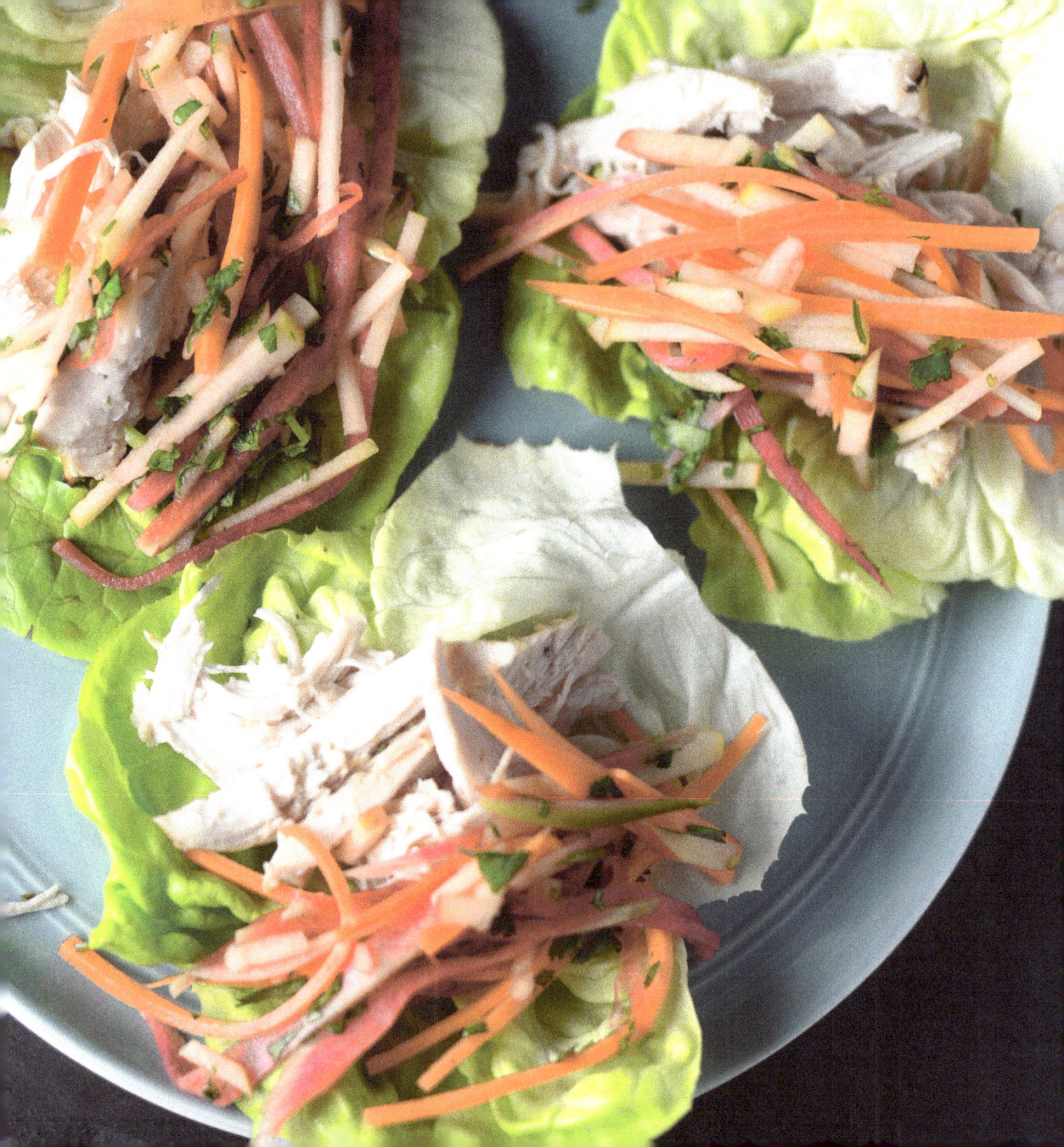

CHICKEN LETTUCE WRAPS

MAKES 6 TO 8 SERVINGS

Okay, lettuce wraps aren't actually a "Beast Bowl," but they could be if they really wanted to, so I couldn't leave them out. Not to mention the Carrot & Apple Slaw is amazing!

Lettuce wraps are a regular part of my meal prep. Because I make bone broth all the time, I often have a bird's worth of shredded chicken in the fridge. Talk about a twofer: I get a week's worth of delicious bone broth and usually a week's worth of protein. These lettuce wraps are one of my favorite uses for that leftover chicken.

INGREDIENTS

- 2 to 3 pounds of cooked shredded chicken (Use leftover chicken if you have it.)
- Butter lettuce leaves
- Carrot & Apple Slaw /135

DIRECTIONS

Pull the lettuce leaves, wash, and then gently dry with a paper towel or a clean kitchen towel.

PRO TIP: You can also use a salad spinner for this step.

Top with shredded chicken and Carrot & Apple Slaw.

Add a little Vietnamese Dressing /140.

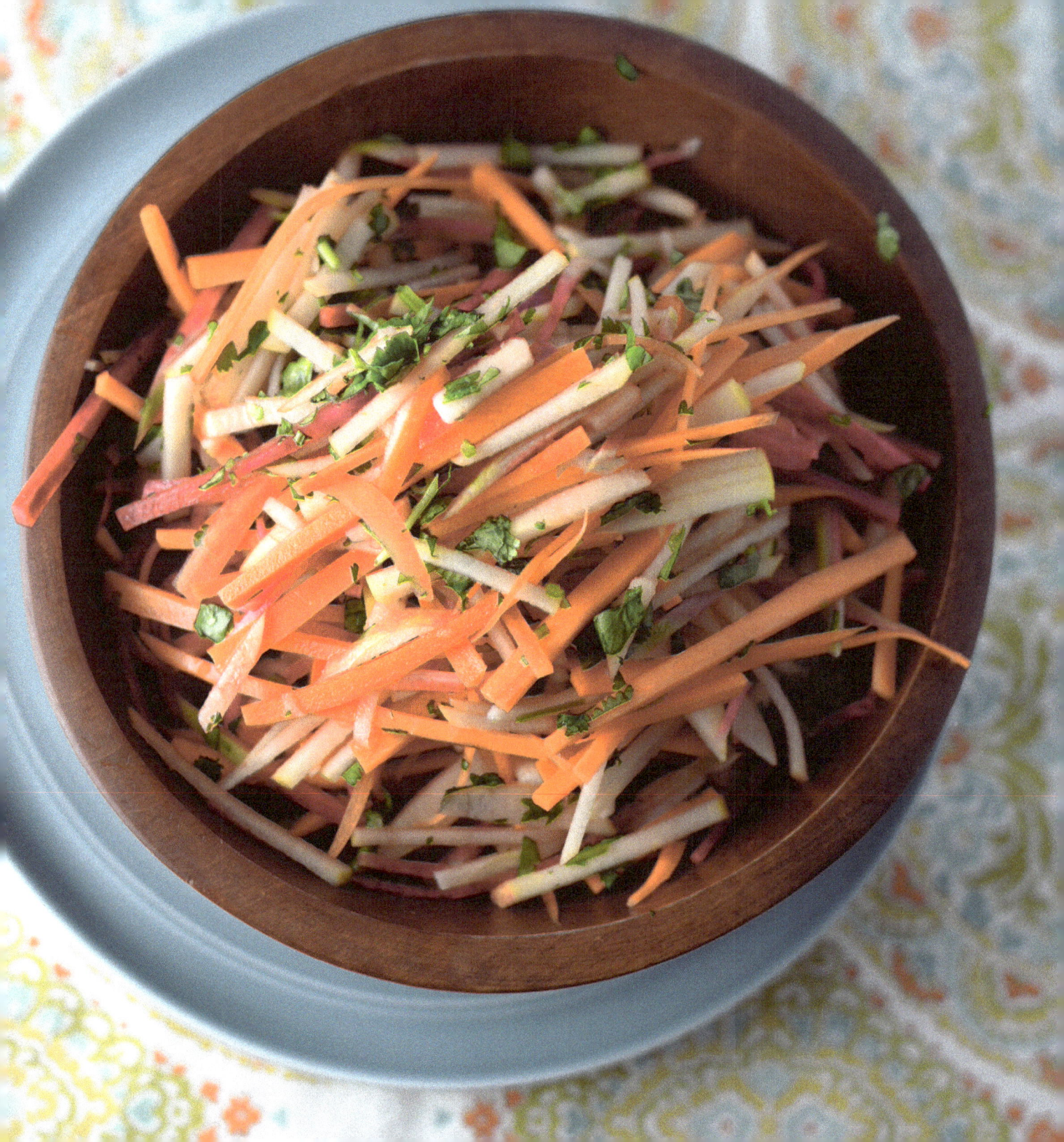

CARROT & APPLE SLAW

INGREDIENTS

2 large carrots, fine julienned (2 to 3 cups)
2 Granny Smith apples, fine julienned (2 to 3 cups)
1 large watermelon radish, fine julienned (½ to 1 cup)
½ bunch cilantro, finely chopped
2 tablespoons rice wine vinegar
1 to 2 teaspoons coconut oil or avocado oil
1 lemon, juiced
½ teaspoon Himalayan sea salt

DIRECTIONS

Peel and cut the carrots, apples, and radishes into matchsticks. Place them in a large nonreactive bowl.

Add the cilantro, rice wine vinegar, coconut oil, lemon juice, and salt.

Toss to coat.

Store in an airtight container for a week.

NOTES

PRO TIP: A mandoline slicer makes quick work of the knife work.

CHAPTER 5
DRESSINGS & SAUCES

Add Some Bling!

Dressings and sauces are the icings on the cake in this world of Beast Bowls. My goal is to give you an arsenal of recipes that you can use in a multitude of ways.

In this chapter, I've tried to provide a dressing for every occasion. You'll even find a few extras that aren't specifically tied to any specific Beast Bowl. Just remember the basic Beast Bowl formula is Protein + Sauce = Yum.

Dressings are really easy to make. They all follow a super simple formula that, once mastered, can be tweaked to fit your favorite flavors. Think outside the bowl. One dressing can be used with a variety of proteins.

BASICS OF VINAIGRETTES

Vinaigrettes are dressings that are built on a base of oil and acid, usually vinegar. The varieties are endless. Making a basic vinaigrette is really easy and way healthier than buying the bottled dressings that have a bunch of preservatives and stabilizers in them. Who wants all that?

You can make vinaigrettes with either a whisk or a Mason jar.

WHISK METHOD

Add everything but the oil to a medium- to large-sized bowl.

Whisk the ingredients together. This is the acid base of the dressing.

Start to slowly drizzle the oil into the acid base. I usually start with about a teaspoon of oil.

Adding the oil slowly while whisking vigorously allows you to build an emulsion. The reason for doing this is that the emulsion will discourage the oil and vinegar from separating. Basically, it gives you a prettier dressing.

MASON JAR METHOD

Add all the ingredients to a Mason jar and shake vigorously. Pour.

PRO TIP: Promptly remove all guests at the table who mention that your dressing is not a proper emulsion!

NOTES ON STORAGE

Store any leftover dressing in the refrigerator for up to a month. Oil may solidify in the colder temperature of your refrigerator. The dressing is still perfectly fine. Simply remove the dressing from the refrigerator and let it come to room temperature before you re-shake and serve.

VIETNAMESE VINAIGRETTE

This umami-ful dressing is the perfect accompaniment to the Lemongrass Shrimp Bowl (53) or the Asian Chicken Meatball Bowl (47).

Vietnamese Vinaigrette can be served with any Asian-style grilled meat and salad. It adds just the right amount of savory flavor and ties together the hot, grilled meat and cold, fresh veggies.

INGREDIENTS

- 2 tablespoons light brown sugar
- 3 tablespoons rice wine vinegar
- 2 limes, juiced
- 3 tablespoons fish sauce, like Red Boat brand
- 1 serrano pepper, quartered lengthwise
- ½ cup cold water

DIRECTIONS

In a small bowl, stir together the brown sugar, vinegar, lime juice, fish sauce, and serrano pepper.

Stir in the cold water and let the mixture sit for 15 minutes.

NOTE

Leftover dressing will keep refrigerated for at least a week.

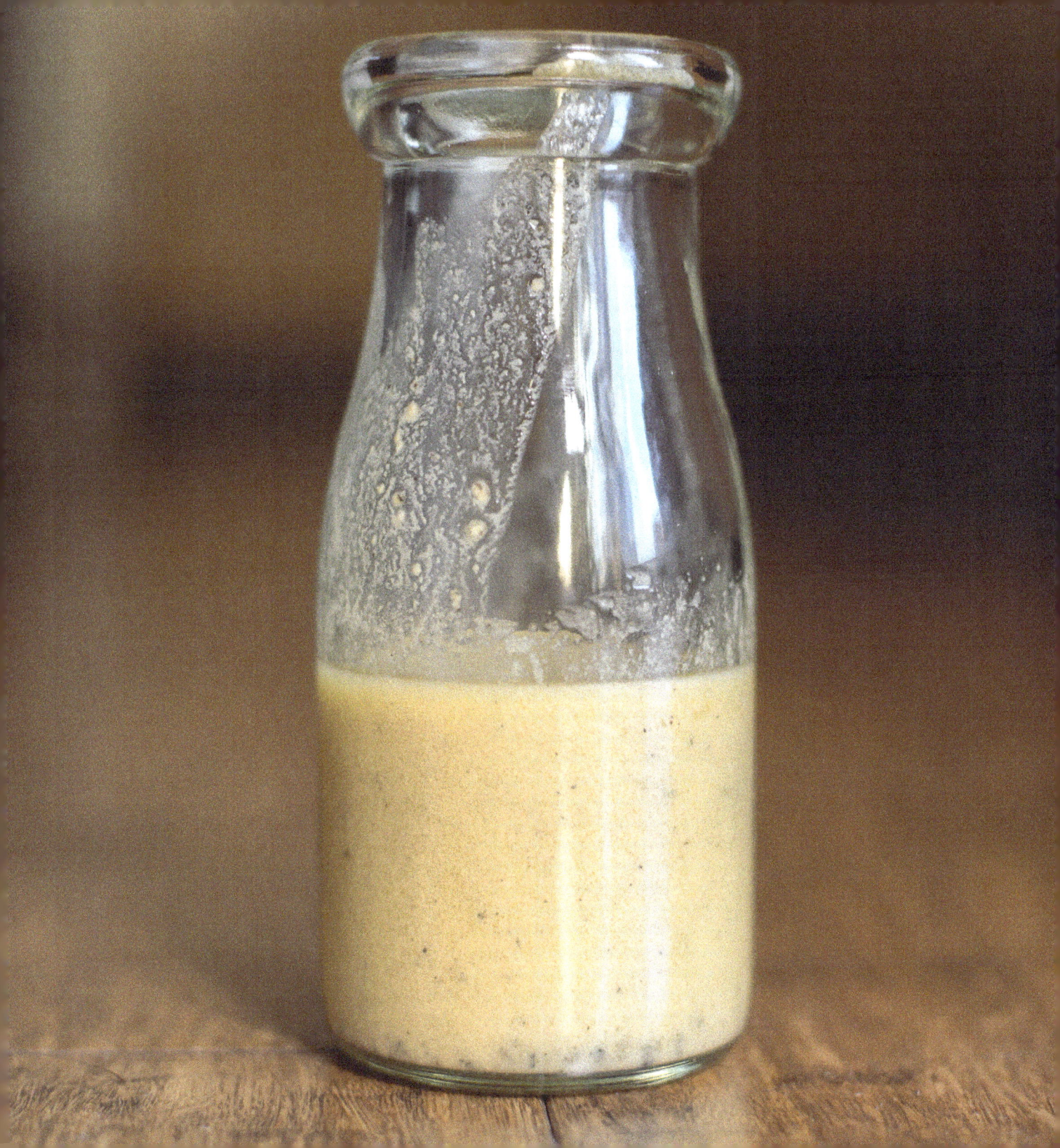

CHAMPAGNE VINAIGRETTE

INGREDIENTS

2 teaspoons Kosher salt
1 teaspoon black pepper
½ cup champagne vinegar
½ cup olive oil

DIRECTIONS

Add the salt, pepper, and vinegar to a bowl.

Whisk.

Add a few drops of olive oil and whisk until emulsified.

Start to add the oil slowly while continuing to whisk vigorously.

CITRUS VINAIGRETTE

INGREDIENTS

1 small shallot, minced
¼ cup champagne vinegar or white wine vinegar
1 lemon, juiced
½ orange, juiced
¼ teaspoons finely grated lemon zest
Kosher salt
Black pepper
¾ cup coconut oil or avocado oil

DIRECTIONS

Add the shallot, vinegar, lemon juice, orange juice, lemon zest, salt, and pepper to a bowl.

Whisk.

Add a few drops of olive oil and whisk until emulsified.

Start to add the oil slowly while continuing to whisk vigorously.

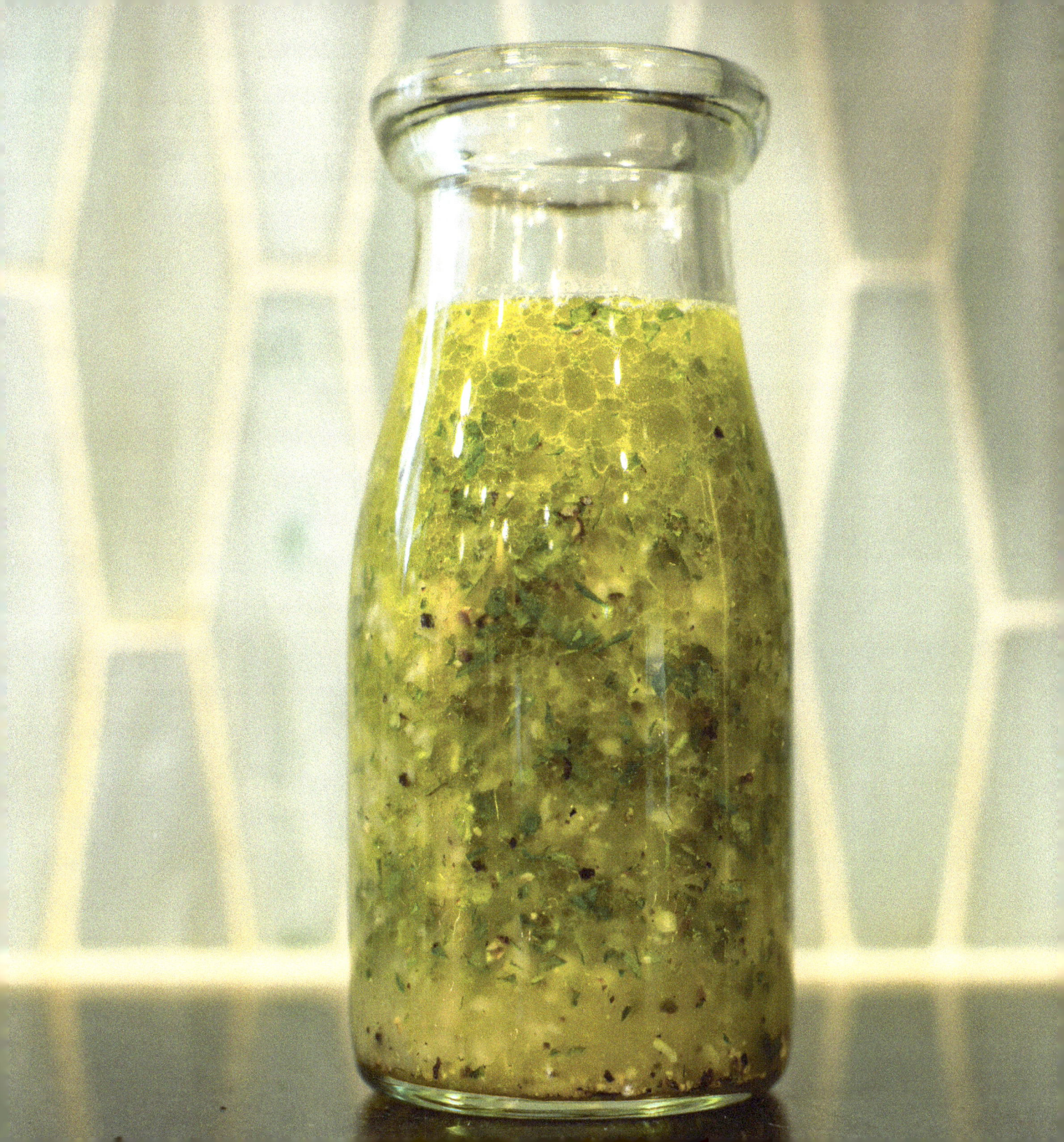

GREEK VINAIGRETTE

INGREDIENTS

2 lemons, juiced
¼ cup red wine vinegar
6 cloves garlic, pressed
1 tablespoon fresh oregano, finely minced
1 teaspoon Kosher salt
¼ teaspoon black pepper
½ cup olive oil
¼ cup crumbled feta (optional)

DIRECTIONS

Squeeze the juice from 2 lemons. Add to a medium bowl.

Add the vinegar to the bowl.

Add the garlic, oregano, salt, and pepper to the liquid. (Use less salt if adding feta.)

Whisk in the olive oil as you drizzle it slowly into the lemon juice.

Stir in the feta, if desired.

HERBES DE PROVENCE VINAIGRETTE

INGREDIENTS

½ cup champagne vinegar
2 teaspoons Kosher salt
1 teaspoon black pepper
2 teaspoons Herbes de Provence Seasoning Mix /185
½ cup olive oil or avocado oil

DIRECTIONS

Add the salt, pepper, seasoning mix, and vinegar to a large bowl.

Whisk.

Add a few drops of olive oil and whisk until emulsified.

Start to add the oil slowly while continuing to whisk vigorously.

MUSTARD VINAIGRETTE

INGREDIENTS

2 teaspoons Kosher salt
1 teaspoon black pepper
2 tablespoons Dijon mustard or brown mustard
½ cup white balsamic vinegar
½ cup olive oil

DIRECTIONS

Add the salt, pepper, mustard, and vinegar to a bowl.

Whisk.

Add a few drops of olive oil and whisk until emulsified.

Start to add the oil slowly while continuing to whisk vigorously.

RED WINE VINAIGRETTE

INGREDIENTS

2 teaspoons Kosher salt
1 teaspoon black pepper
½ cup red wine vinegar
½ cup olive oil

DIRECTIONS

Add the salt, pepper, and vinegar to a bowl.

Whisk.

Add a few drops of olive oil and whisk until emulsified.

Start to add the oil slowly while continuing to whisk vigorously.

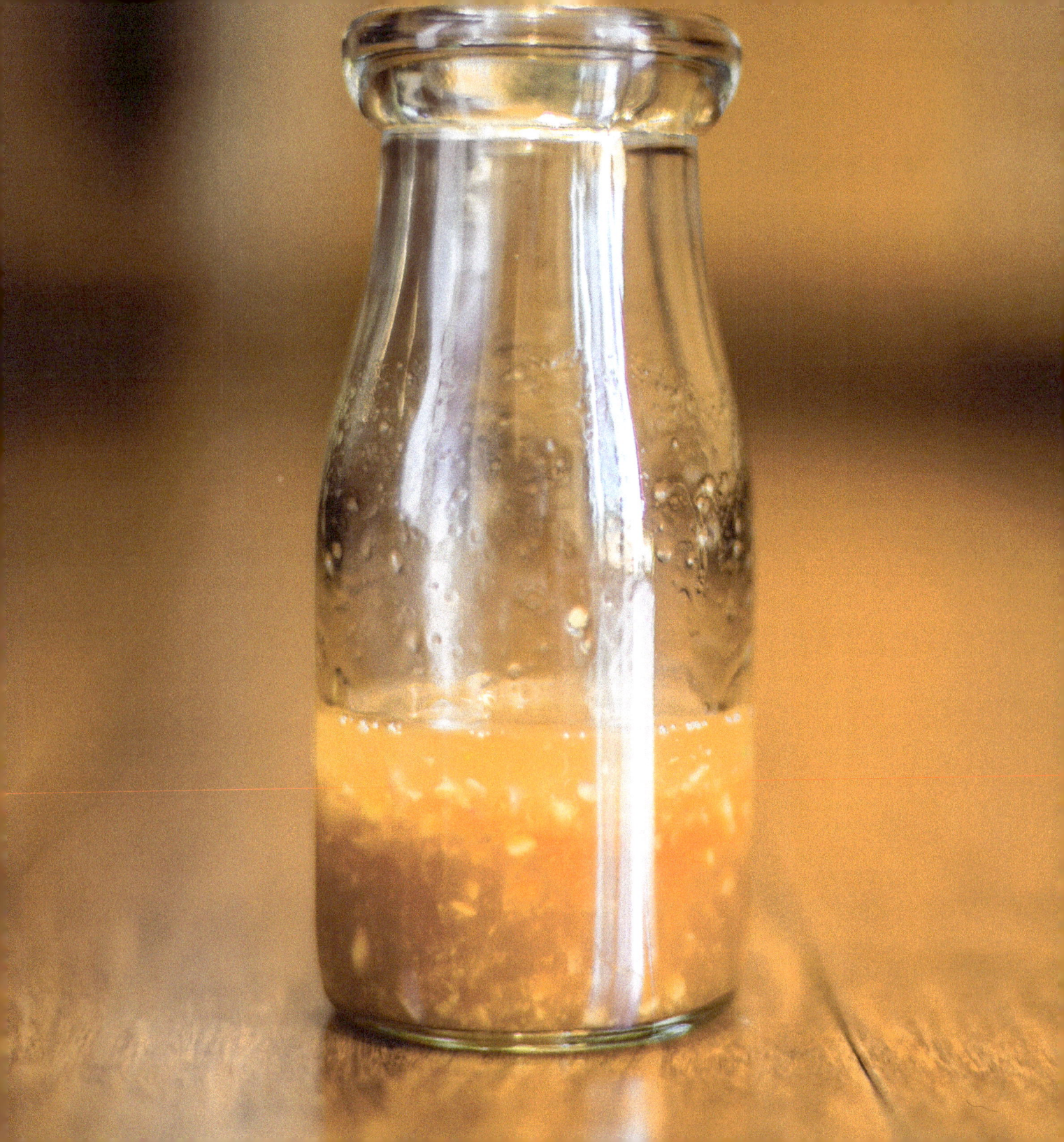

SESAME GINGER VINAIGRETTE

INGREDIENTS

2 tablespoons shallot, minced
4 teaspoons fresh ginger, grated
4 cloves garlic, pressed
4 tablespoons soy sauce or tamari
½ cup seasoned rice wine vinegar
2 tablespoons honey
2 tablespoons water
1 teaspoon sesame oil
½ cup coconut oil

DIRECTIONS

Add all the ingredients except the coconut oil to a medium bowl.

Whisk.

Add a few drops of coconut oil and whisk until emulsified.

Start to add the oil slowly while continuing to whisk vigorously.

TOMATO BALSAMIC VINAIGRETTE

INGREDIENTS

2 tablespoons shallot, minced
1 tablespoon Dijon mustard
2 teaspoons tomato paste
¼ cup balsamic vinegar
¼ cup olive oil

DIRECTIONS

Add the shallots, Dijon mustard, tomato paste, and vinegar to a bowl.

Whisk.

Add a few drops of olive oil and whisk until emulsified.

Start to add the oil slowly while continuing to whisk vigorously.

BASICS OF MAYO

Mayonnaise is built with the same oil + acid, just like a vinaigrette, + egg yolks. The proteins in the egg yolk allow you to build that creamy texture that you know and love in all your favorite creamy-style dressings. The ranch dressings in this chapter all start with a basic mayo plus seasonings.

Once you learn the basics, you can tweak these dressings to fit in with anything that you're serving. Because mayonnaise has only a few simple ingredients, it's important to pick the absolute best ingredients that you can find.

Fresh, homemade mayonnaise is a fantastic source of healthy fats because you'll use high-quality eggs, a great source of Omega-3s. Then you'll complement these eggs with a flavorful and Omega-3-rich oil.

Remember that the dietary fats you eat are used as building blocks and incorporated directly into your cells during the cell regeneration process. Knowing this gives me the incentive to use the best fats I can find when cooking.

THE 3 BASIC COMPONENTS OF MAYONNAISE:

1. EGGS

Use the freshest eggs that you can find. I like to choose eggs that are pasture-raised. Whenever possible, look for eggs from local sources. The best eggs are from chickens that are able to forage on insects. You know that you have a really nutritious egg if you crack it open and the yolk is a deep yellow, nearly orange color. These eggs are both rich in flavor and full of healthy Omega-3s.

2. ACID

The acid component of mayonnaise gives it a brightness of flavor. For the basic recipe in this book, you will use about 2½ tablespoons of acid.

CITRUS-BASED ACIDS

Citrus-based acids can be used to create a dressing that can be matched to whatever flavor profile you are trying to create. My favorites include lemon juice, lime juice, orange juice, and grapefruit juice.

VINEGAR-BASED ACIDS

White vinegar is lightly flavored and comes in almost any flavor that you can image. Experiment and find your favorite flavor combos. Some of my favorites include lemongrass and pomegranate. The two that I keep in the refrigerator at all times are champagne vinegar and red wine vinegar.

3. OIL

My absolute favorite is avocado oil. It has a mild flavor that blends well with a number of different spice combinations that I like to use. Alternatively, olive oil can be used to create a stronger flavored mayonnaise. The rich olive flavor is a great complement to Mediterranean-style spices. Listed below are just a few suggestions. (Stay away from really strong-flavored oils and vegetable oils, which are highly refined.)

My go-to oils for dressings: avocado oil, walnut oil, and macadamia nut oil.

MAKE YOUR OWN MAYO!

Making your own mayonnaise is super easy! I like making my own mayo for two reasons. First, it allows me to pick and choose the flavors that go into it. Once you master the basic mayo recipe, you can get creative and add different spices. Second, it's ridiculously cost-effective. Many of the gourmet mayos in the store that can easily run in the $8 range. I've even seen an avocado oil-based mayo for $11.

Do yourself a favor and learn this simple kitchen skill — you will be glad that you did! You can make mayo by hand with a whisk, or you can also use a food processor (fitted with a metal blade) or an immersion blender.

USING A WHISK

Add the egg yolk and dry ingredients to a glass bowl.

Whisk in your acid (vinegar or citrus juice).

While whisking briskly, start to add the oil a few drops at a time.

The mixture will start to thicken as it becomes emulsified.

Once you have an emulsion, you can start to add the oil in a slow stream while continuing to whisk.

Continue adding oil until your mayo is the right consistency for whatever you will be using it with. (You may use less or more oil than the recipe calls for.)

For salad dressings, the mayo can be thinner. For dips or spreads, you may prefer it a little thicker. Thicker mayo will require more oil than thinner mayo.

Practice makes perfect here. Once you get a feel for how the emulsion comes together, it's easy! If your dressing ends up on the looser side, it'll still be delicious.

USING A POWER TOOL

Add all the ingredients except the oil to a high powered blender or food processor, or use an immersion blender.

With the machine running, start adding oil, slowly at first.

Once the mixture is emulsified, you can stream oil into the machine.

Continue to add oil until the mayo reaches the desired thickness.

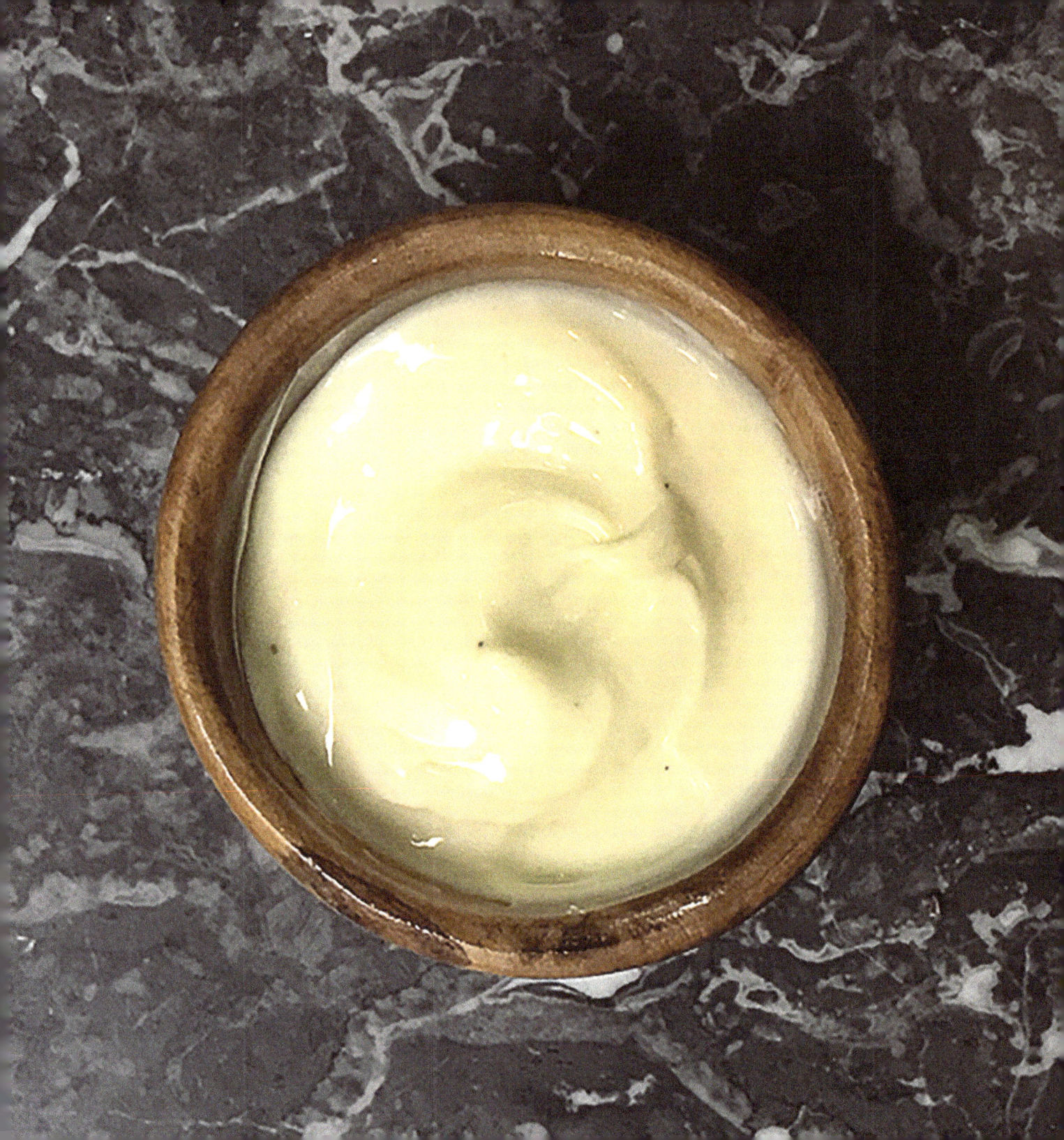

BEASTASTIC MAYO

Mastering homemade mayo is easy. If it sounds intimidating at first, give it a try anyway. It's just a few egg yolks and a squeeze of lemon juice. You can totally do that. Then you just add oil slowly. Bam! Mayo. And it's way better for you than the stuff from the store.

My two favorite types of oils to use in this recipe are macadamia nut oil and avocado oil. Both have a really mild flavor, which allows you to use this base with all different kinds of seasoning. This mayo is the perfect canvas for the mayo-based sauces that you will find in the rest of this chapter.

INGREDIENTS

2 egg yolks
1 teaspoon Kosher salt
½ teaspoon dry mustard powder
1 lemon, juiced
⅓ to 1 cup oil (depending on how thick you want the mayo)

FOOD PROCESSOR / HAND BLENDER DIRECTIONS

Add the eggs, salt, and mustard to a food processor.

Turn the machine on high.

With the machine running, add about half the acid.

Continue to keep the machine running and start to add the oil. Add about 1 teaspoon of oil to start an emulsion.

Continue to add oil by drizzling it into the bowl.

Once the mixture comes together as a creamy emulsion, add the rest of the acid.

Continue to add the oil until the mixture is the thickness that you want. This can vary depending on how you will use this mayo.

Enjoy it plain or add spices to season up your mayonnaise.

NOTES

ALTERNATIVE: Use the whisk method. /150

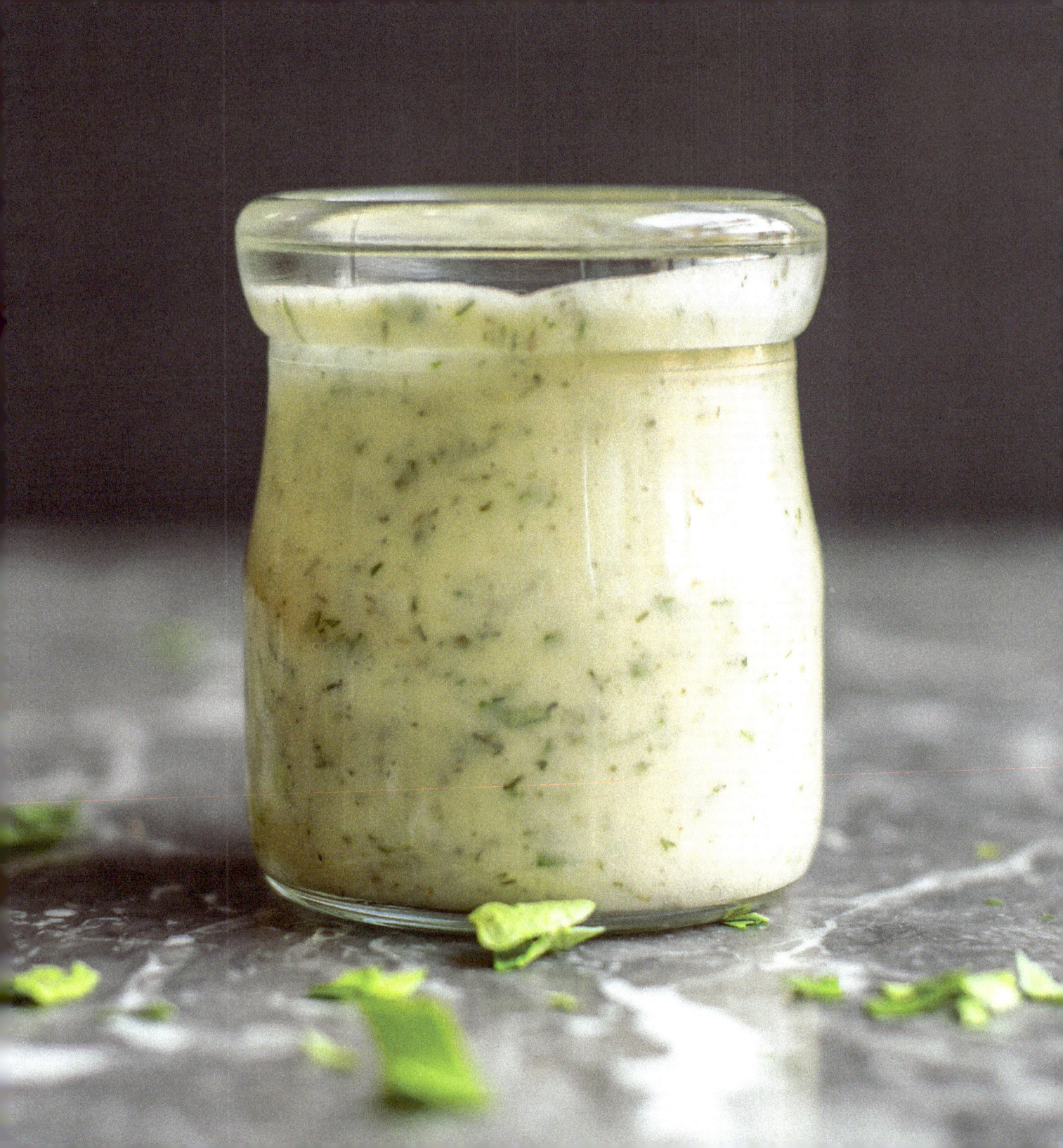

PALEO RANCH

Ranch dressing is an iconic staple for all things dipping related. From carrots to hot wings, ranch dressing just seems to make everything taste better.

This ranch dressing is dairy-free and made with healthy fats so you can enjoy it and feel good about it, too. I created this recipe to pair with the Fried Chicken Beast Bowl, and it is fantastic with that. This recipe is also great on any salad, and it's a perfect dipping sauce for any roasted potato.

INGREDIENTS

- 1 egg yolk
- 1 teaspoon dried dill
- ½ teaspoon dry mustard powder
- ½ teaspoon onion powder
- 2 teaspoons fresh parsley
- ½ teaspoon Kosher salt
- 1 lemon, juiced
- 1 cup macadamia nut oil or any mildly flavored light oil
- ½ cup coconut milk

DIRECTIONS

Add the egg yolk and dry ingredients to a glass bowl.

Whisk in the lemon juice or vinegar.

Whisking very briskly, start to add the oil, a few drops at a time.

The mixture will start to thicken as it becomes emulsified.

Once you have an emulsion, you can start to add the oil in a slow stream while continuing to whisk.

Continue adding oil until your mayo is the right consistency for whatever you will be using it with. (You may use less or more oil than the recipe calls for.)

NOTES

ALTERNATIVE: Use the power tool method. /151

BUFFALO RANCH

Buffalo Ranch is a spicier version of the traditional Paleo Ranch dressing recipe. I like to make this dressing on the thinner side by adding a little less oil or thinning with a little water at the end. Then I serve it as a dressing with the Buffalo Beast Bowl.

My second favorite way to eat this is with the Roasted Potatoes. I spice them up with the Mediterranean Seasoning Mix and then use this as a dip.

INGREDIENTS

- 1 egg yolk
- 1 tablespoon champagne vinegar or lemon juice
- ¼ teaspoon dried dill
- ¼ teaspoon garlic powder
- ¼ teaspoon onion powder
- ¼ teaspoon paprika
- ⅛ teaspoon cayenne pepper
- ½ teaspoon Kosher salt
- ⅛ teaspoon black pepper
- ½ cup avocado oil or walnut oil

DIRECTIONS

Using a high powered blender or food processor, blend the egg and vinegar.

With the machine still running, add the spices.

Then, with the machine still running, slowly drizzle in the avocado oil. Blend until the mixture is emulsified.

CHIPOTLE RANCH

Chipotle Ranch is everything a burrito bowl could ask for. It's spicy and zesty and pairs incredibly well with the Chipotle Chicken Beast Bowl and Mom-Style Taco Beast Bowl. This is my absolute favorite dipping sauce for sweet potato fries.

Once you get the hang of making your own homemade salad dressings, you will seriously wonder why you ever bought them in the first place.

INGREDIENTS

- 1 egg yolk
- 1 tablespoon champagne vinegar or lemon juice
- 1 to 2 canned chipotle peppers or 2 teaspoons dried chipotle pepper
- 2 teaspoons Taco Seasoning Mix
- 2 tablespoons hot sauce, like Chipotle Cholula brand
- ½ lime, juiced
- ½ cup avocado oil

DIRECTIONS

Using a high powered blender or food processor, blend the egg and vinegar.

With the machine still running, add the spices and hot sauce.

Then, with the machine still running, slowly drizzle in the avocado oil.

Blend until the mixture is emulsified.

BEAST SAUCE

INGREDIENTS
¾ cup mayonnaise
¼ cup ketchup
1½ tablespoons yellow mustard
¼ cup sweet pickle relish

DIRECTIONS
Whisk all the ingredients together.

LOUIE DRESSING

INGREDIENTS
1 cup mayonnaise
¼ cup chili sauce
½ lemon, juiced

DIRECTIONS
Whisk all the ingredients together.

GARLICKY AIOLI

INGREDIENTS

1 egg
4 cloves garlic, pressed
½ lemon, juiced
½ cup macadamia nut oil or light olive oil
½ teaspoon Kosher salt
¼ teaspoon black pepper

DIRECTIONS

Whisk the egg, garlic, and lemon juice together.

Add a few drops of oil.

Whisk, then add a little more oil, very slowly at first, while whisking continuously.

Continue to add oil slowly while whisking vigorously.

Add salt and pepper to taste.

REMOULADE

INGREDIENTS

1 cup mayonnaise
2 tablespoons Dijon mustard
2 teaspoons whole grain mustard
½ lemon, juiced
1 tablespoon Louisiana-style hot sauce
1 teaspoon Worcestershire sauce
2 cloves garlic, minced
2 teaspoons capers, roughly chopped
1 tablespoon flat-leaf parsley, finely chopped
1 green onion, finely chopped
1 teaspoon mild paprika
¼ teaspoon Kosher salt
⅛ teaspoon cayenne pepper

DIRECTIONS

Whisk all the ingredients together.

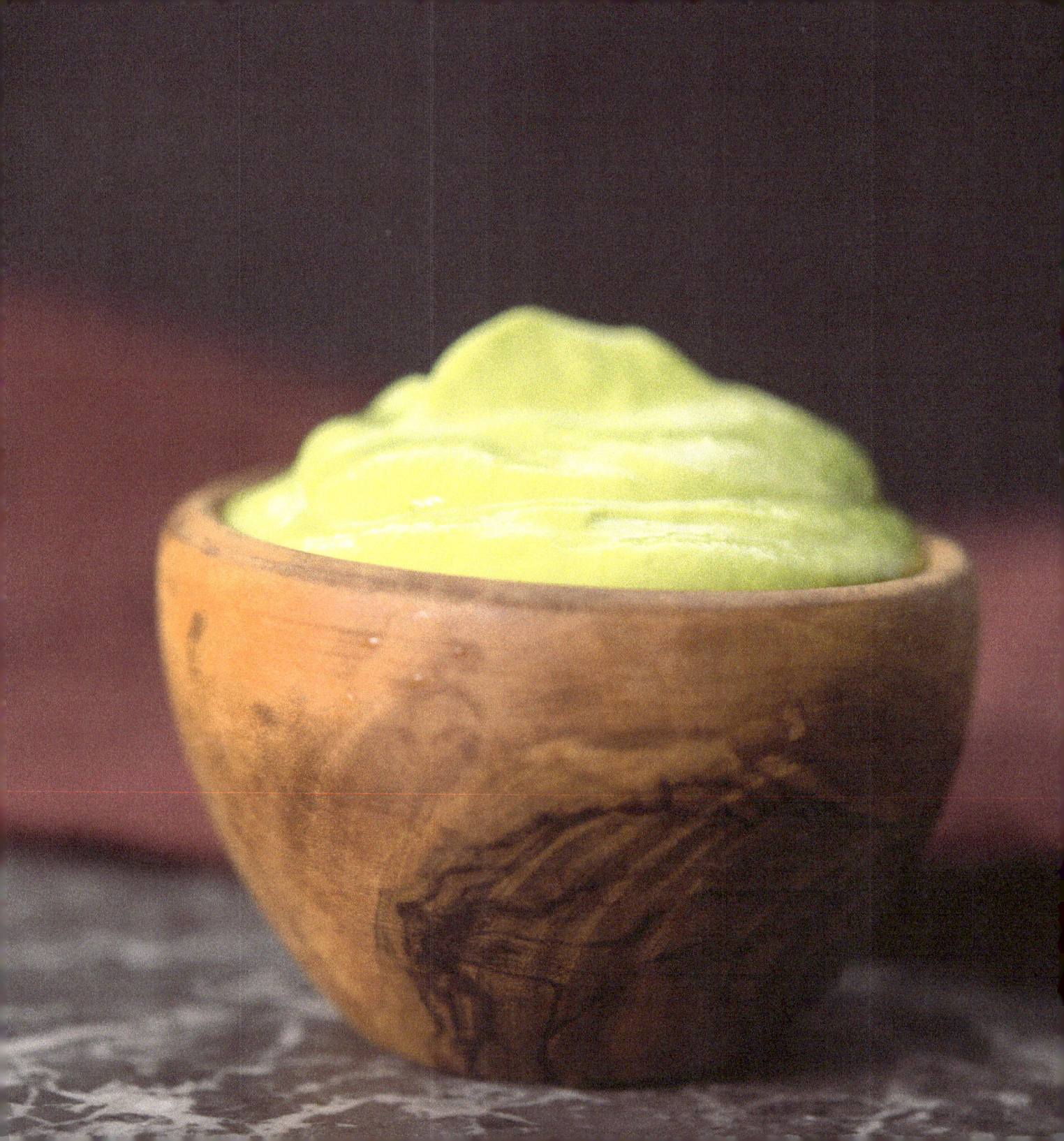

AVOCADO CILANTRO LIME CREMA

This zesty avocado crema is cool and creamy! It adds a smooth and cooling flavor to the spiciest Beast Bowls, tacos, or burritos. I even enjoy this crema on eggs.

Cremas come together in just a few minutes and add so much flavor to everything you add them too!

INGREDIENTS

½ cup crème fraiche or sour cream
½ avocado
½ bunch cilantro, finely chopped
½ lime, juiced

DIRECTIONS

Add all the ingredients to a high powered blender or food processor.

Blend until smooth.

Add salt and pepper to taste.

Serve on top of your favorite tacos or taco salad.

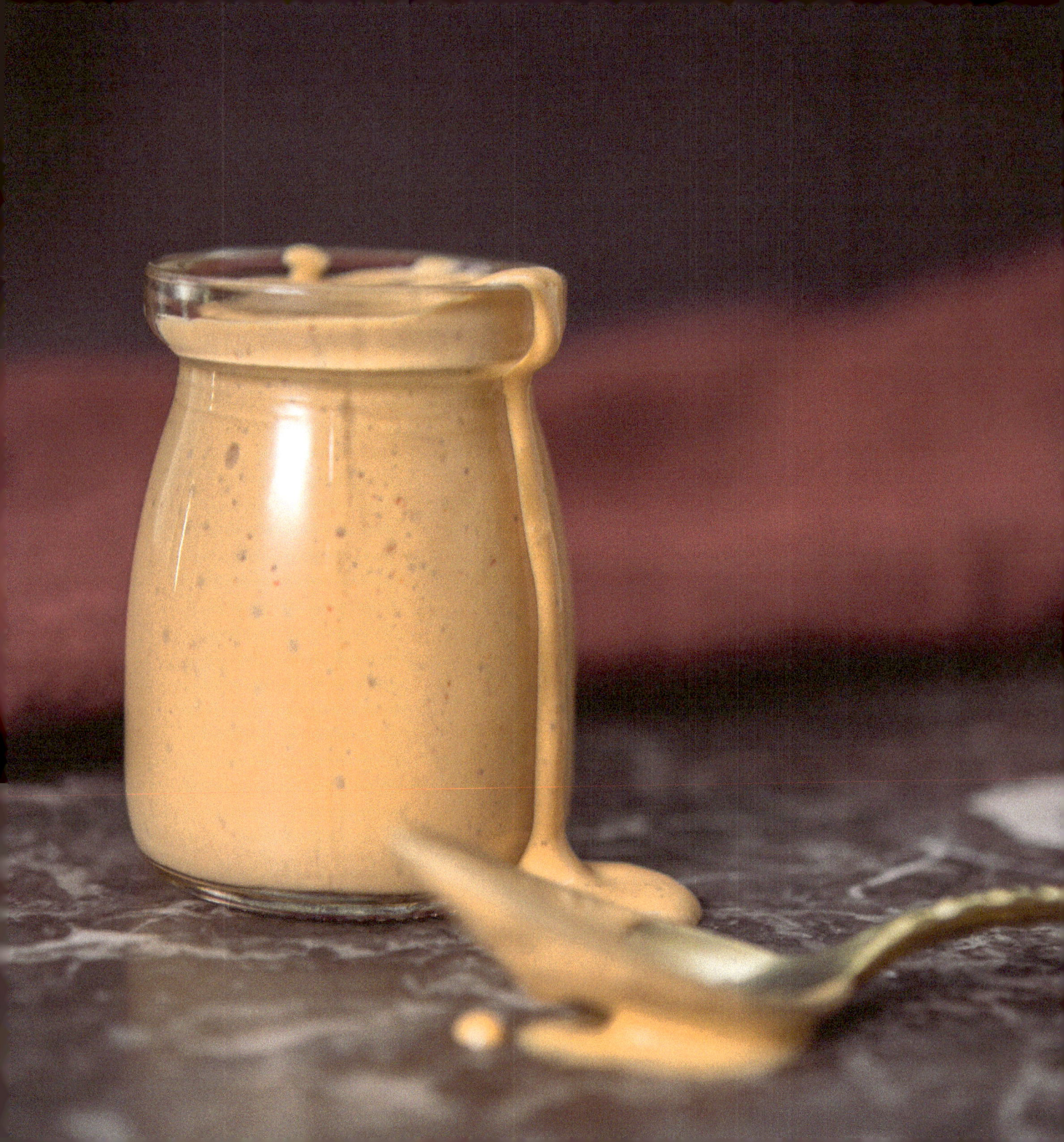

CHIPOTLE CREMA

This spicy crema is perfect on every kind of protein – it's the perfect complement to the Chipotle Beast Bowl, and of course, your tacos will thank you! I especially love this crema with steak.

With just a quick whirl of your blender or food processor, this is sure to become your new favorite sauce!

INGREDIENTS

1 cup sour cream or crème fraiche
2 to 3 whole chipotle peppers

DIRECTIONS

Add all the ingredients to a high powered blender or food processor.

Blend until smooth.

Add salt and pepper to taste.

Serve on top of your favorite tacos or taco salad.

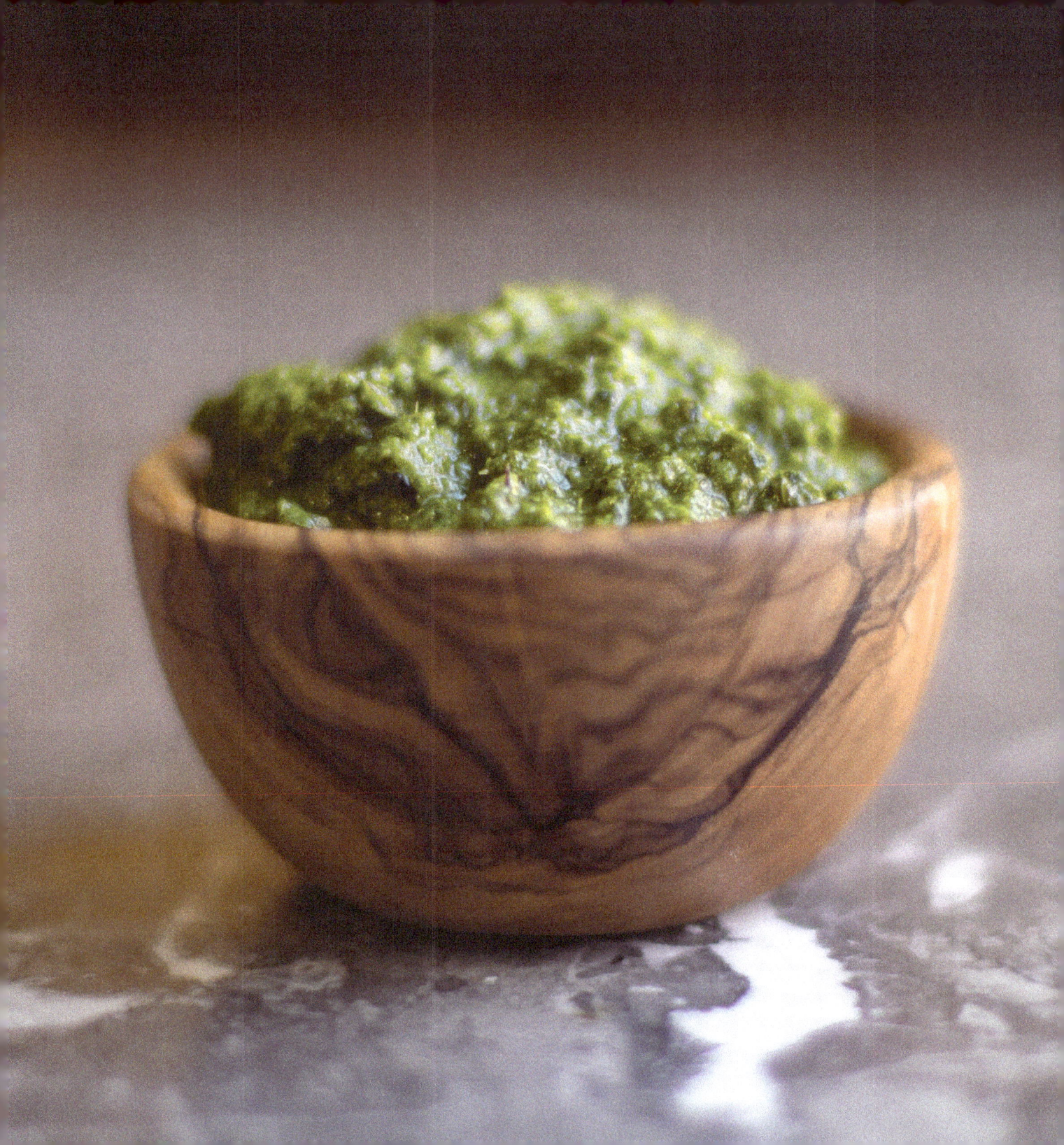

CHIMICHURRI SAUCE

Chimichurri Sauce is a fresh, spicy condiment that is delicious on all grilled or roasted meats and vegetables. Some of my favorite ways to eat this zesty green condiment are slathering it on grilled flat iron steak or adding a fat dollop onto a plateful of roasted root vegetables.

INGREDIENTS

- 4 jalapeño peppers, seeded and coarsely chopped
- ½ bunch green onions
- ⅓ cup shallots
- ¼ bunch cilantro
- 2 tablespoons sherry vinegar
- ¾ teaspoon Kosher salt
- ½ teaspoon black pepper

DIRECTIONS

Add all the ingredients to a food processor.

Pulse until the ingredients are finely minced.

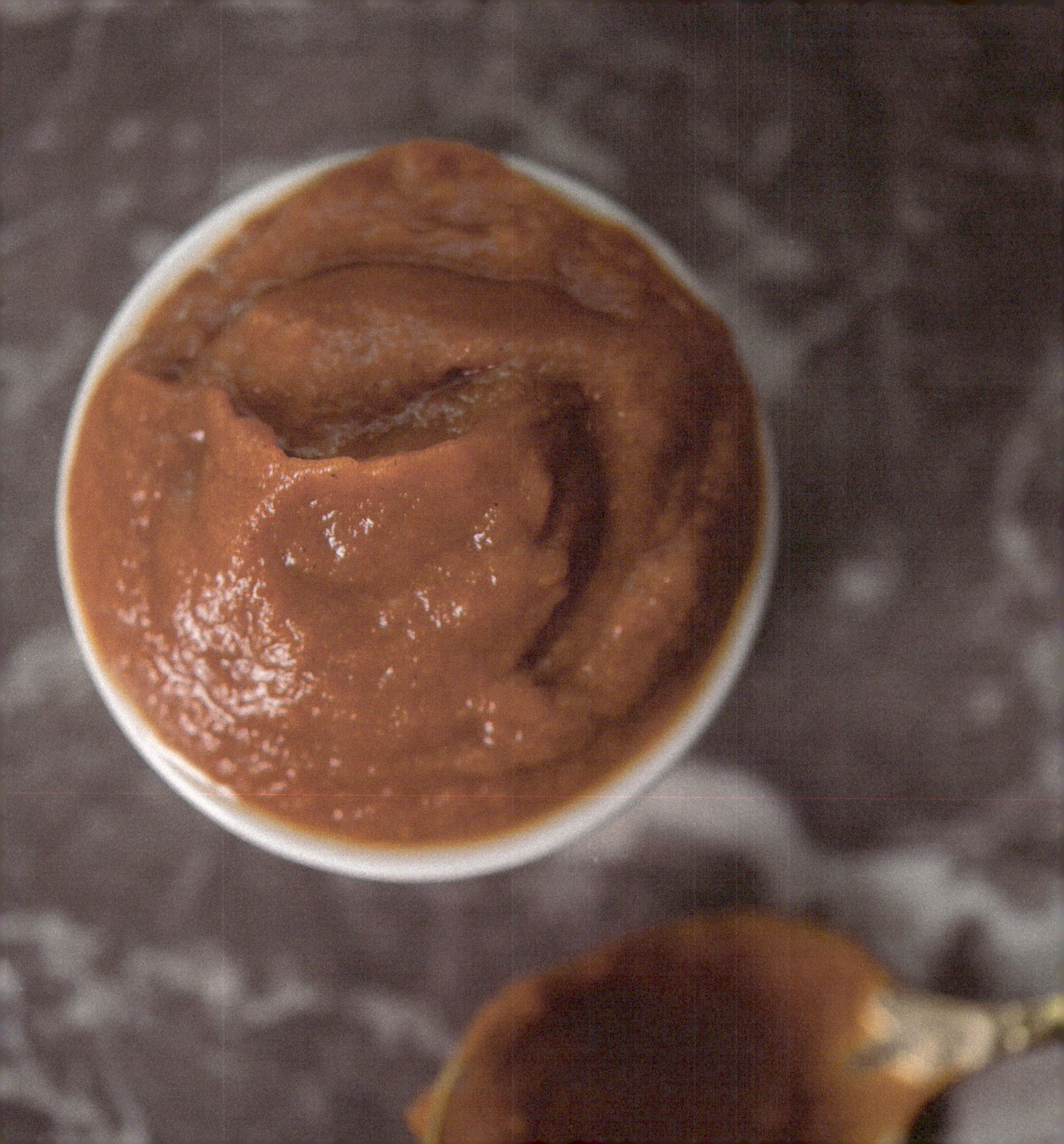

PALEO KETCHUP

Ahh, good old ketchup. You can eat it on everything, but it's usually full of sugar. Make it from scratch — it tastes even better than the sweet stuff! Try the spiced up chipotle version with some sweet potato fries. The chili version is delicious with roasted Yukon Gold potato fries.

Try them both and find your favorite.

INGREDIENTS

- 1 28-ounce can tomato puree
- 2 tablespoons tomato paste
- 4 tablespoons apple cider vinegar or white vinegar
- ¾ to 1 cup carrots, shredded
- 1 teaspoon garlic powder
- 1 teaspoon onion powder
- ½ teaspoon allspice
- 1 teaspoon Kosher salt
- 4 tablespoons maple syrup
- 2 tablespoons water, to thin

DIRECTIONS

Add all the ingredients to a blender.

Blend until smooth.

Store for up to 2 weeks in an airtight container in the refrigerator.

NOTES

CHIPOTLE VERSION: Add 1 to 2 chipotle peppers.

SPICY CHILI VERSION: Add 1 to 2 tablespoons of chili sauce.

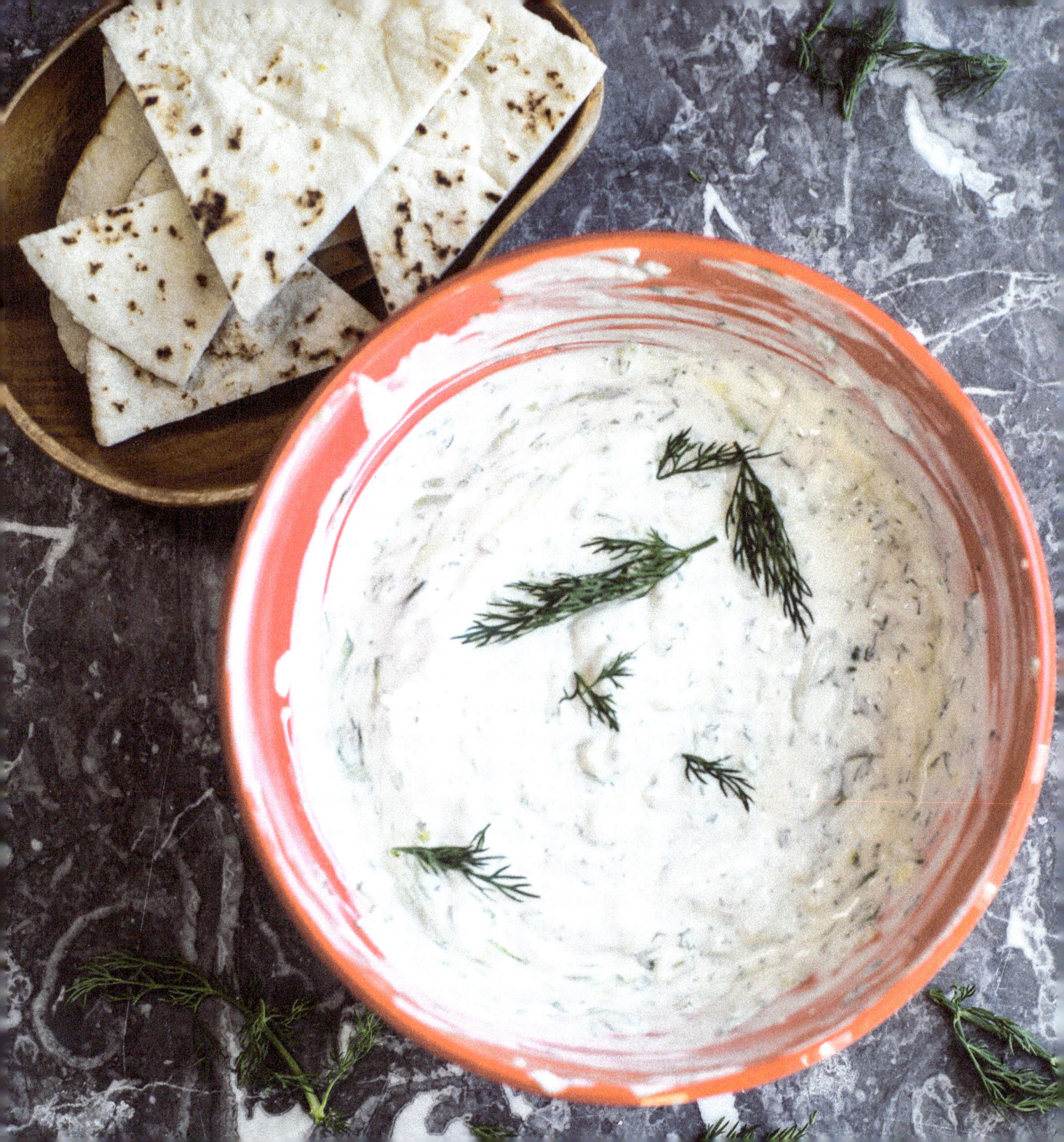

TZATZIKI

Tzatziki is a traditional Greek condiment that tastes good on absolutely everything. This sauce is amazing with the lamb burgers from the Greek Lamb Burger Beast Bowl. It's also fantastic with roasted veggies like eggplant and carrots.

You can serve it with toasted pita or just add a dollop to a Greek salad.

INGREDIENTS

- 1 cup cucumber, diced or shredded
- 1 to 2 teaspoons of Kosher salt for salting cucumbers
- 2 cups full-fat Greek yogurt
- 3 cloves garlic, minced
- 3 teaspoons fresh dill
- ½ lemon, juiced
- 1 tablespoon olive oil
- 1 teaspoon Kosher salt, adjust to taste
- ¼ teaspoon black pepper

DIRECTIONS

Finely dice or shred the cucumber and place it in a mesh strainer. Sprinkle with salt. Toss and set it aside.

NOTE: This step pulls the excess water out of the cucumber and keeps the tzatziki from getting watery.

Mix the yogurt, garlic, dill, lemon juice, olive oil, salt, and pepper.

Press the liquid out of the cucumbers and then add them to the yogurt mixture.

PRO TIP: Place the cucumbers in a clean kitchen towel, wrap tightly, and squeeze the excess water out.

Add salt and pepper to taste.

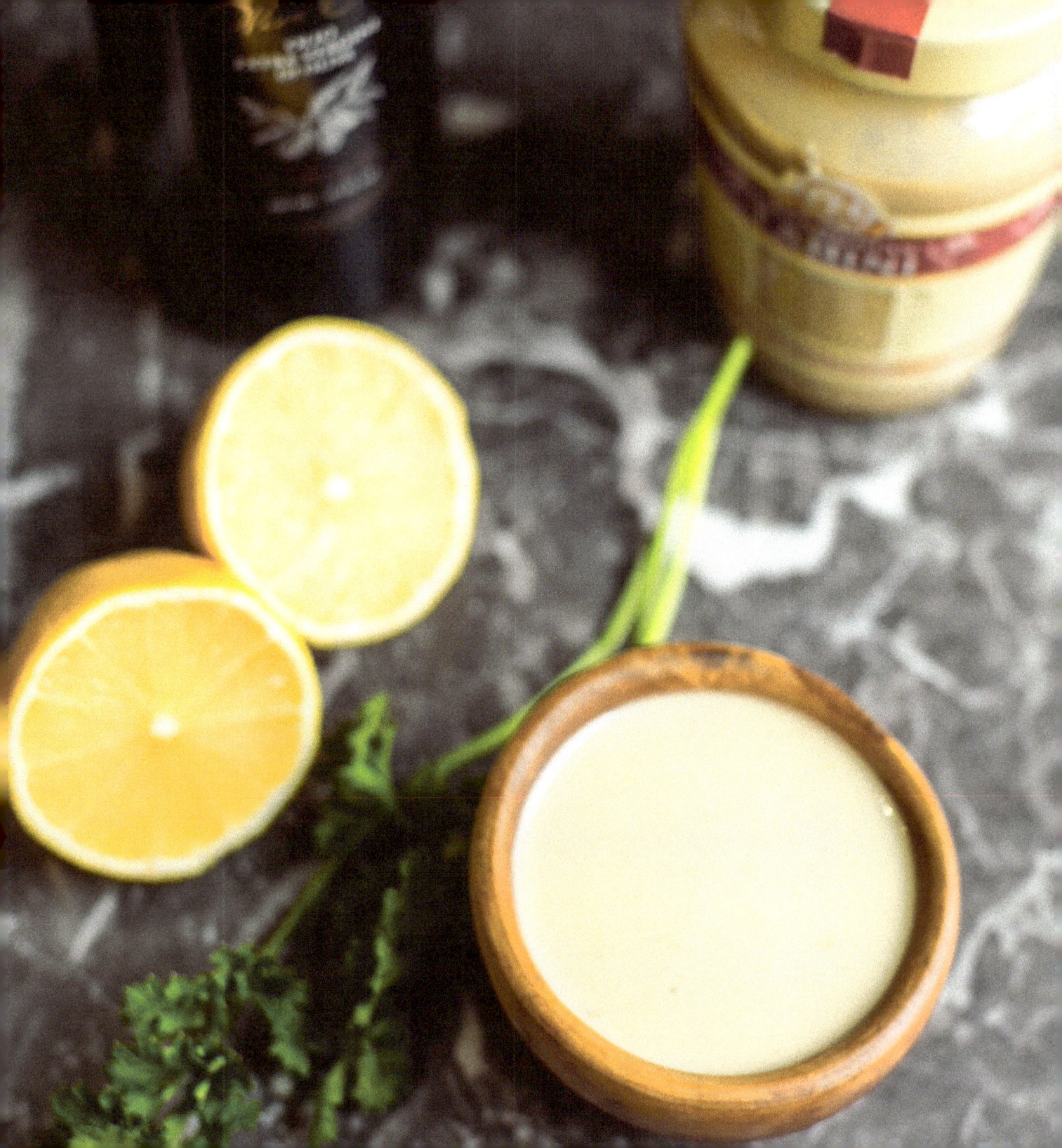

LEMON TAHINI DRESSING

Lemon Tahini Dressing is a super versatile sauce. It can be used as a salad dressing alone, and it's absolutely delicious served with roasted meats and vegetables. I always make a double batch of this dressing. You are sure to go through it quickly.

INGREDIENTS

¼ cup tahini
2 lemons, juiced
¼ cup olive oil
¼ cup water, to thin
1 teaspoon Kosher salt, adjust to taste

DIRECTIONS

Add the ingredients to a medium bowl and whisk until combined.

Add water to thin to the desired consistency.

NOTE: You might not use all the water.

Add salt to taste.

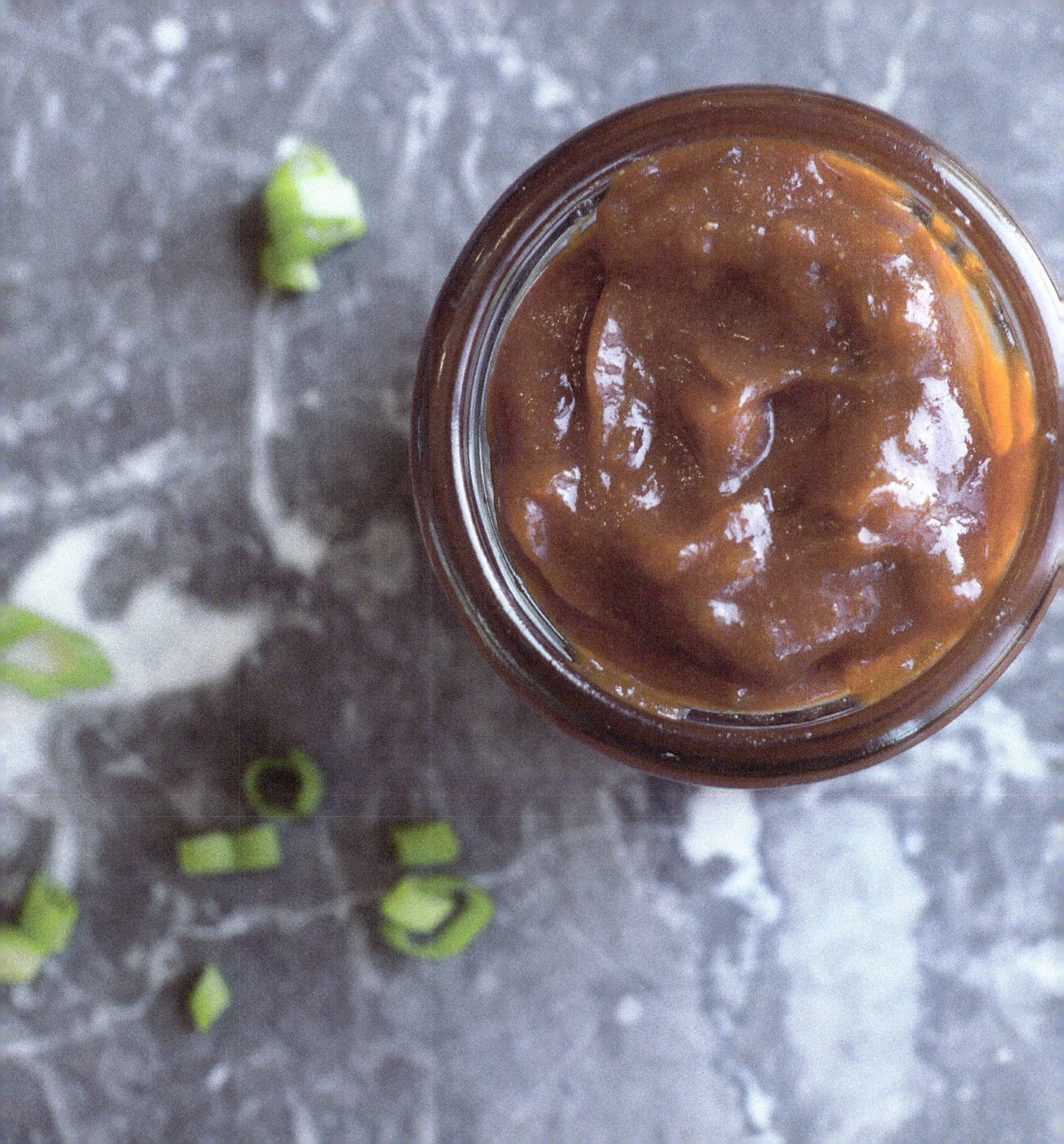

SPICY TANGY BARBECUE SAUCE

Scrap the overly-sugary bottled stuff and try one of these recipes!

This barbecue sauce has been in my family for as long as I can remember. It is a recipe saved from a long-time family friend. I spiced it up with a few jalapeños — there is no doubt that I like to keep things spicy. If you want a less spicy sauce, feel free to leave out the jalapeños.

INGREDIENTS

- 2 tablespoons butter or coconut oil
- ¼ sweet onion, diced
- ¼ cup carrot, finely diced
- ½ cup celery, finely diced
- 1 to 2 jalapeños, finely diced
- 2 tablespoons brown sugar or panela sugar
- 2 tablespoons sherry vinegar
- 1 tablespoon Worcestershire sauce
- 1 lemon, juiced
- 1 cup ketchup
- 1 teaspoon dry mustard powder
- 1 teaspoon Kosher salt

DIRECTIONS

Heat the butter on medium-high in a large saucepan.

Add the onion, carrot, celery, and jalapeños.

Sauté on medium-high until the veggies are tender and fragrant, about 5 minutes.

Add the brown sugar, sherry vinegar, and Worcestershire sauce and stir to combine. Scrape the pan to incorporate all the brown bits.

Add the lemon juice and ketchup, and bring to a simmer.

Reduce the temperature and add mustard and salt to taste.

Add water to thin to the desired consistency.

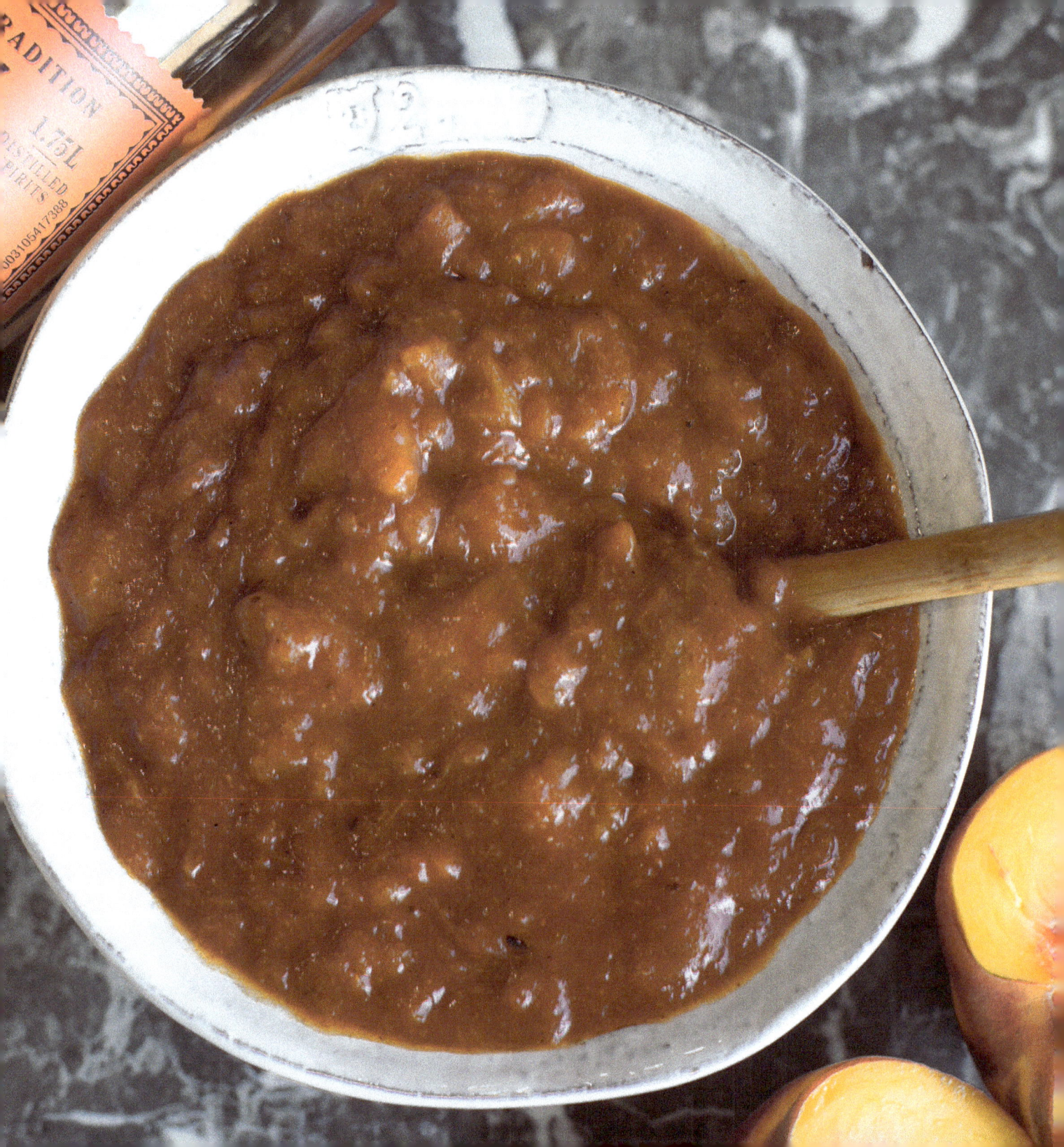

PEACH BOURBON BARBECUE SAUCE

This barbecue sauce is one of a kind. It's saucy and rich with the natural sweetness and mellow flavor of ripe summer peaches paired with a nice bourbon. What could be better?

I originally created this recipe to go with my Grilled Pork Skewers, which you can find on the blog at FoodologyGeek.com. I wanted to add it here so that you have another way to eat your Pulled Pork Beast Bowl. The barbecue sauce is sure to be a favorite. It is so bomb on grilled chicken, too!

INGREDIENTS

2 teaspoons coconut oil
½ medium onion, finely diced
2 cloves garlic, pressed
4 yellow peaches, peeled and diced
¼ cup tomato paste
½ cup panela sugar or brown sugar
½ cup bourbon
3 tablespoons apple cider vinegar
¼ teaspoon allspice
¼ teaspoon cinnamon
½ teaspoon dry mustard powder
½ teaspoon smoked paprika
2 teaspoons Kosher salt
¼ teaspoon cayenne pepper

DIRECTIONS

Add the coconut oil, onion, garlic, and peaches to a medium-sized saucepan.

Cook on medium-high heat until the peaches are soft. Time will vary depending on the ripeness of the peaches.

Add the tomato paste and sugar. Cook until the sugar is dissolved.

Add the bourbon and apple cider vinegar. Bring to a boil.

Reduce the temperature and add the spices.

Simmer to let the spices infuse into the sauce.

Add a little water to thin to the desired consistency, if needed.

Add salt to taste.

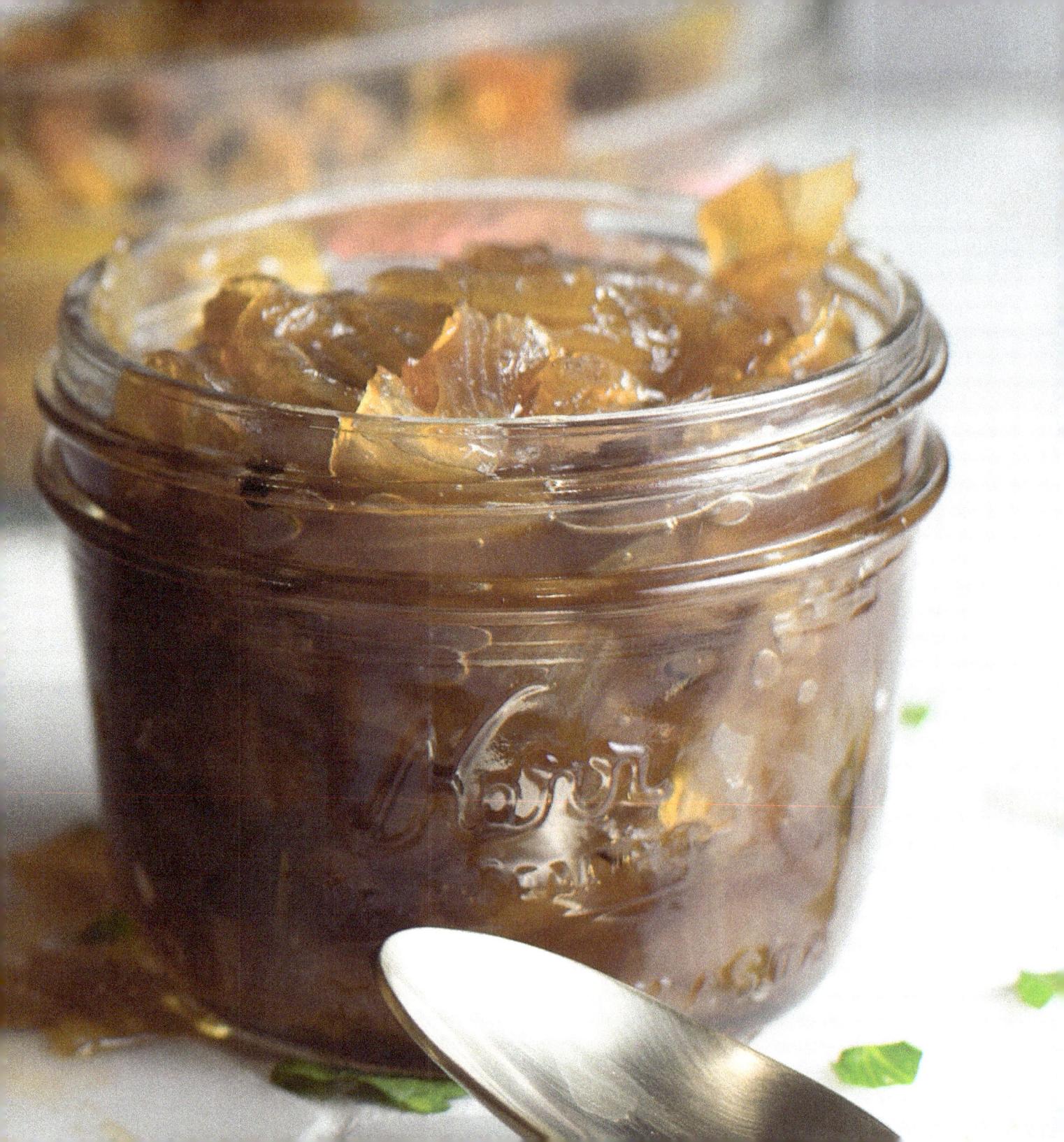

ONION JAM

If you've never tried onion jam, you are in for a treat. Of course this goes with meatloaf! But imagine it on a great burger or on the All-American Burger Beast Bowl.

The other most incredible way to serve this jam is to place it on top of a round of triple cream brie and bake until warm and melty. Serve this with your favorite crackers.

INGREDIENTS

¼ cup coconut oil
3 large sweet onions, cut into ¼ inch dice
2 parsley sprigs
2 bay leaves
1 rosemary sprig
1 cup sugar
¾ cup white balsamic vinegar
½ teaspoon Kosher salt

DIRECTIONS

In a large pot, heat the coconut oil until it is shimmering.

Add the onions and cook them over medium-high heat, stirring occasionally until golden brown, about 15 minutes.

Tie the parsley, bay leaves, and rosemary together with kitchen twine.

Add the herb bundle to the diced onions and cook over low heat, stirring a few times, until fragrant, about 3 minutes.

Sprinkle the sugar over the onions and cook without stirring until the sugar melts, about 5 minutes.

Increase the heat to high and cook without stirring until an amber-brown caramel forms, about 6 minutes.

Stir in the white balsamic vinegar and simmer over low heat, stirring a few times until the jam is thick, about 5 minutes.

Remove and discard the herb bundle.

Season the jam with salt and let it cool.

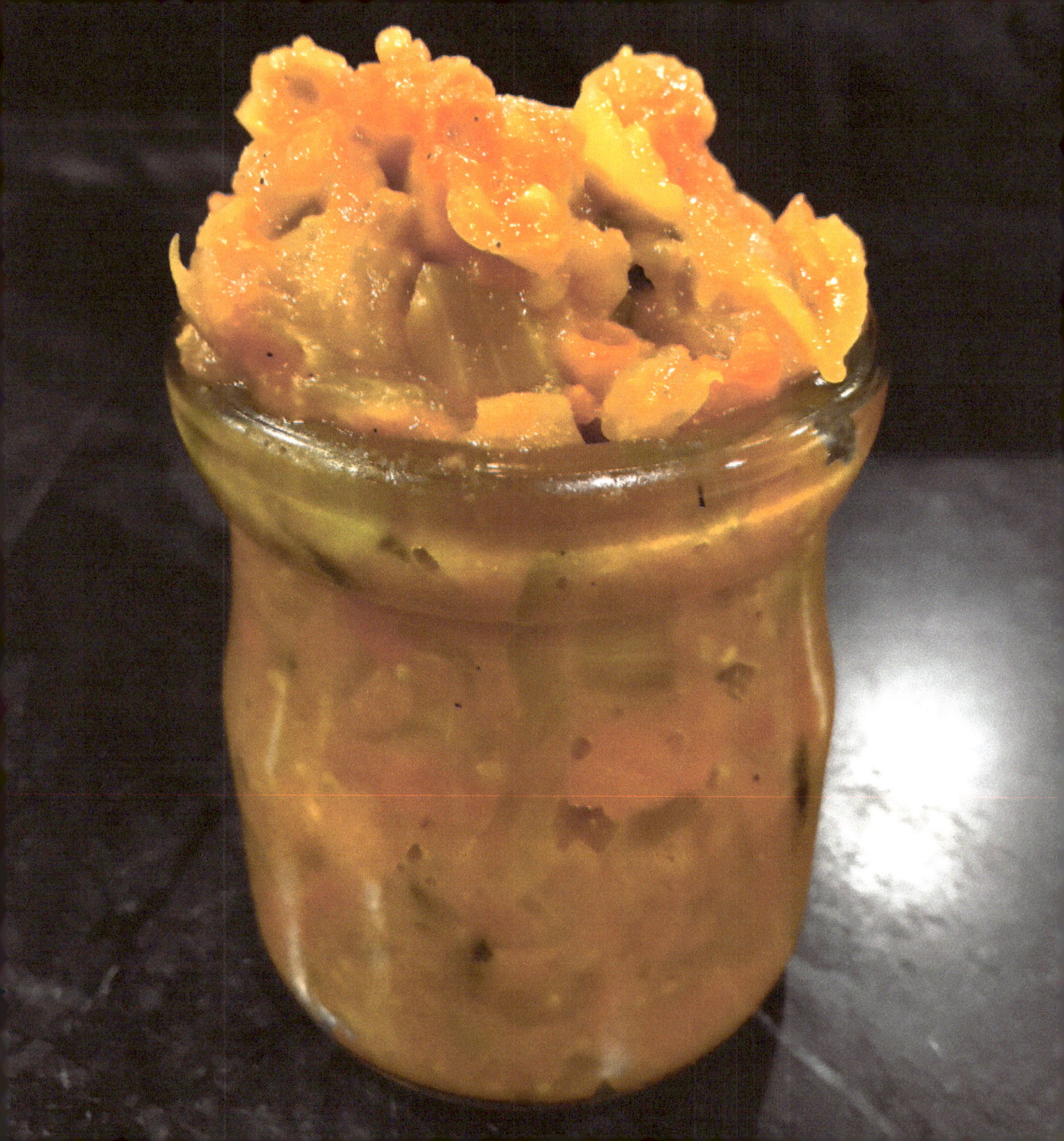

SPICY TOMATO JAM

I used some golden heirloom tomatoes that I had growing in my garden when I made this version of the Spicy Tomato Jam, so don't be alarmed if your jam is red.

Tomato jam is really just a chunky version of ketchup. It tastes amazing with the Paleo Meatloaf Beast Bowl. Substitute tomato jam for ketchup on any burger and you're in for a real treat. Pair it with the onion jam and you get a spicy-sweet flavor combo that will rock your world.

INGREDIENTS

- 1 28-ounce can whole peeled tomatoes, drained
- 2 tablespoons coconut oil
- 1 yellow onion, thinly sliced
- 1 clove garlic, thinly sliced
- 1 teaspoon cumin
- 1 teaspoon curry powder
- 1 teaspoon yellow mustard seeds
- 1 teaspoon sherry vinegar
- ¼ cup fresh oregano, roughly chopped
- 1 teaspoon granulated sugar
- 1 teaspoon Kosher salt
- ½ teaspoon black pepper

DIRECTIONS

Heat the coconut oil to medium-high heat in a medium saucepan.

Add the onions and garlic and sauté until fragrant, about 3 to 4 minutes.

Add the tomatoes. Pour the liquid into the saucepan, and then crush the tomatoes by hand before adding them to the pan.

ALTERNATIVE: Use canned crushed tomatoes.

Add the spices and bring to a boil.

Cover and simmer until the tomatoes are soft and the texture of the sauce is like a chunky jam.

Serve with meatloaf or burgers.

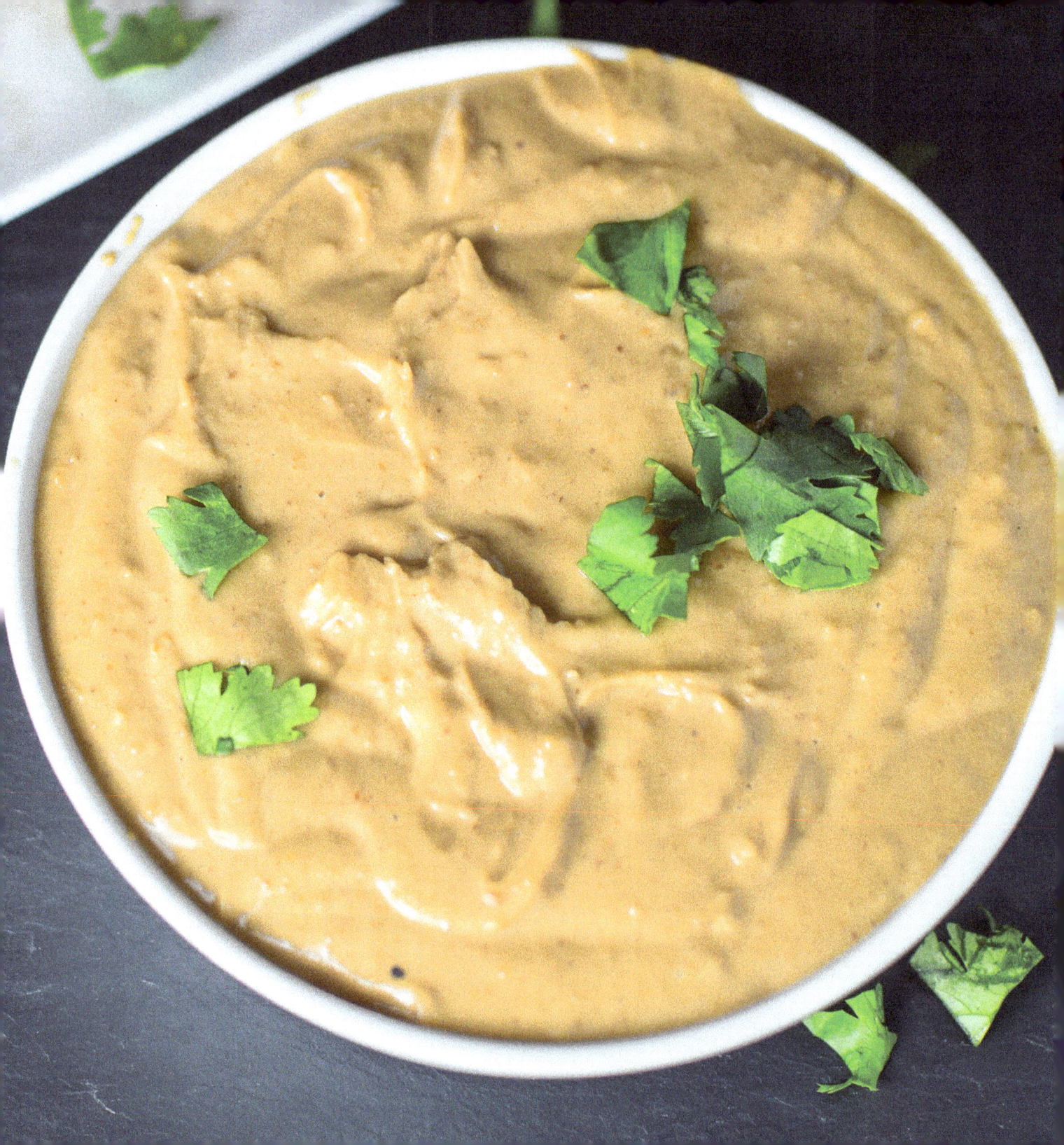

SATAY PEANUT SAUCE

INGREDIENTS

½ cup smooth peanut butter
2 tablespoons soy sauce or tamari
1 clove garlic, pressed
1 teaspoon fresh ginger, grated
1 teaspoon crushed red pepper
3 tablespoons coconut milk or coconut cream
2 tablespoons cilantro, finely chopped
2 tablespoons water, to thin

DIRECTIONS

Whisk all the ingredients together until smooth and well combined.

Add water to thin to the desired consistency.

NOTES

PRO TIP: Stabilized peanut butter works best here. You know, the one that doesn't have the oil separating out.

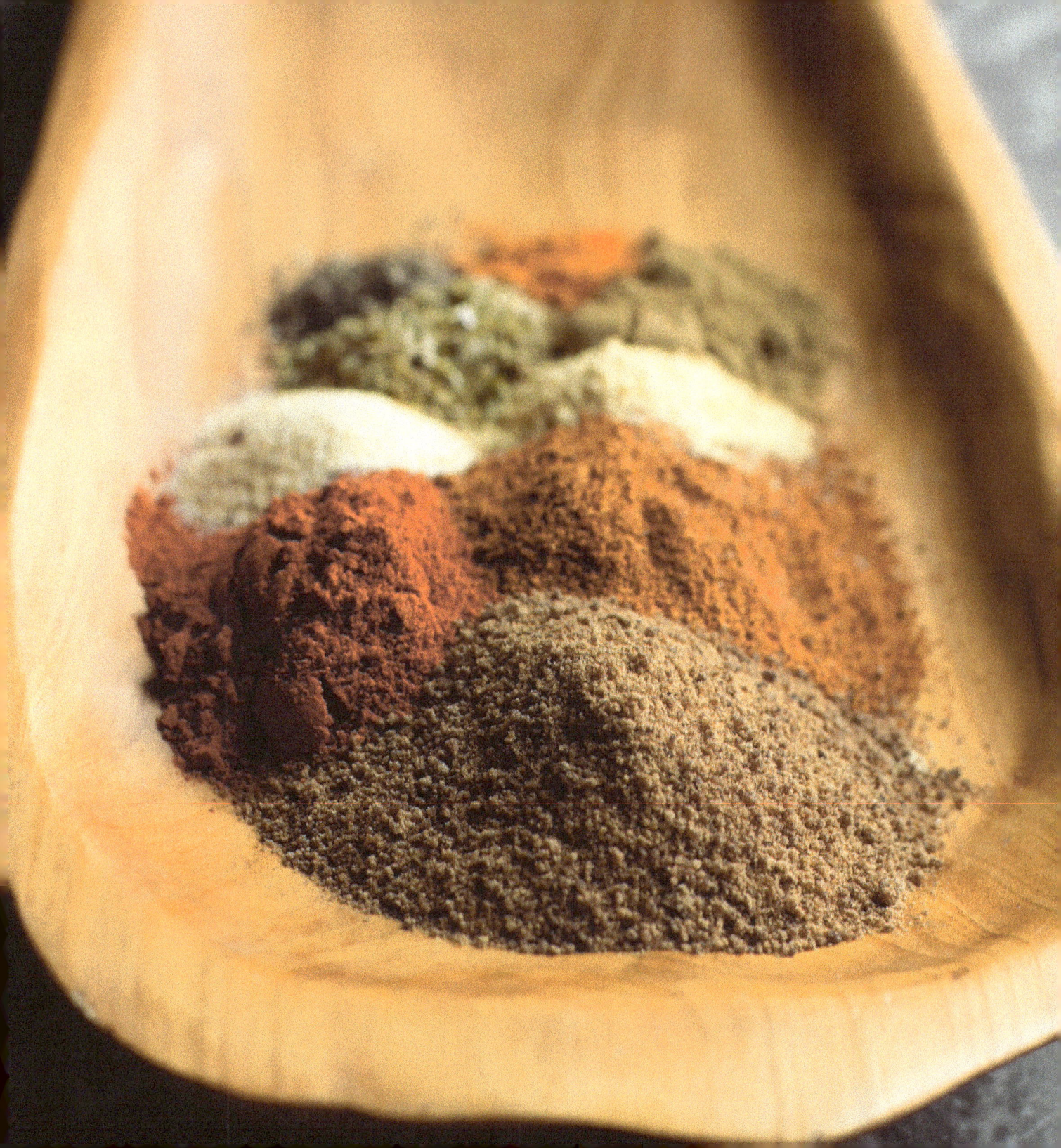

CHAPTER 6
SEASONINGS

Pull Into Flavor Town

Seasoning mixes are the secret weapon for quick and easy meal prep! These tasty gems make it effortless to give your protein a serious flavor punch. Having a batch of these mixes around makes it easy to create a food snob-worthy meal in no time at all.

Most of these recipes make about a half a cup. Store them in clip top glass jars, and they'll keep for months. Don't forget to label them, so they're easy to find in the spice cabinet.

MEDITERRANEAN

This particular seasoning mix can be used on absolutely everything: fish, shrimp, tofu, chicken, roasted potatoes, or vegetables. Double this recipe and store it in an airtight container so that you'll always have some on hand. This mix is probably the most used seasoning mix in our house.

- 1 tablespoon cumin
- 3 tablespoons dried oregano
- 3 tablespoons sesame seeds
- 1 tablespoon Kosher or Himalayan salt
- 1 tablespoon crushed red pepper flakes (use less if you like it less spicy)

HERBES DE PROVENCE

This seasoning is ideal on roasted chicken and in chicken salad. Imagine chicken salad with homemade mayo and a few teaspoons of Herbes de Provence mixed in. Put it on a really nice piece of toasted sourdough, and it's magic! This seasoning also makes a great Herbes de Provence Vinaigrette.

- 1 tablespoon dried lavender flowers, lightly ground
- 1 tablespoon dried marjoram
- 1 tablespoon dried sage
- 1½ tablespoons dried savory
- 3 tablespoons dried tarragon
- ½ teaspoon dried orange zest (optional)

BUFFALO

Cook up an entire bag of thawed chicken tenderloins or cleaned tail-on shrimp, add your favorite hot wing sauce, chop up a big stack of carrots and celery, and then toss on some Buffalo Ranch Dressing. And of course, use this mix when you make the Buffalo Chicken Beast Bowl.

3 tablespoons garlic powder
3 tablespoons onion powder
3 tablespoons paprika
1 tablespoon Kosher salt
2 teaspoons black pepper
2 teaspoons cayenne pepper

PUMPKIN PIE SPICE

This is my grandma's pumpkin pie spice mix. I use this in place of all commercial pumpkin pie spice. This is absolutely fantastic on roasted sweet potatoes. A few teaspoons with some Kosher salt, coconut oil, and maple syrup make a warm and comforting side.

7 tablespoons cinnamon
2 tablespoons ground cloves
5 tablespoons ground ginger
2 tablespoons nutmeg

BARBECUE RUB

Use this rub on chicken, pork, steak, and shrimp. Throw a pork shoulder in the slow cooker or Instant Pot. You don't even need to add any liquid in the slow cooker. Just rub a 4-lb pork shoulder with about 4 tbsp and then let it cook on low all day.

The second tastiest way to use this rub is on roasted sweet potatoes. Barbecue spiced sweet potato fries + Chipotle Ranch Dressing = HEAVEN.

¼ cup chili powder
½ cup coconut sugar
2 teaspoons cumin
1 tablespoon garlic powder
1 tablespoon dry mustard powder
2 teaspoons dried oregano
¼ cup smoked paprika
¾ teaspoon black pepper
½ to 2 teaspoons cayenne pepper

JAMAICAN JERK

This spicy island flavor is so good on chicken. It is delicious on chicken wings, but it's equally amazing as a rub on chicken breasts or thighs.

1 teaspoon allspice
¼ teaspoon cinnamon
1 tablespoon garlic powder
½ teaspoon nutmeg
2 teaspoons onion powder
1 teaspoon paprika
2 teaspoons dried parsley
2 teaspoons sugar
2 teaspoons dried thyme
2 teaspoons Kosher or Himalayan salt
½ teaspoon black pepper
2 teaspoons cayenne pepper
½ teaspoon crushed red pepper

TACO

This is the second most used spice in the collection. It works best on chicken, beef, pork, and shrimp. Use this to give a batch of browned ground beef and onions bomb-tastic flavor! Toss it on top of some Mexican Slaw. Talk about super easy lunch prep.

2½ tablespoons chili powder
2 teaspoons coriander
1½ teaspoons cumin
2 teaspoons onion powder
1 tablespoon dried oregano
2 teaspoons paprika
1½ teaspoons Kosher or Himalayan salt
¼ teaspoon black pepper
1 to 3 teaspoons cayenne pepper

CHAPTER 7
SNACKS

What You Crave

We all need a little bit of sweetness in our lives. Keeping true to the philosophy of real food for real, I've created some of my favorites treats right here!

I don't believe in counting calories. I think that eating should be a joyous celebration that makes you happy and nourishes your body from a place of love. When you live in a state of deprivation, you aren't living a full life. When you don't let yourself have the really good stuff, you feel an unhealthy craving for all the things you shouldn't eat. Which often leads to overeating it.

These snacks are wholesome and made with high-quality ingredients. They are meant to satisfy your sweet tooth, whether you are in the mood for something crunchy, or something chocolatey. Indulge and feel good about it!

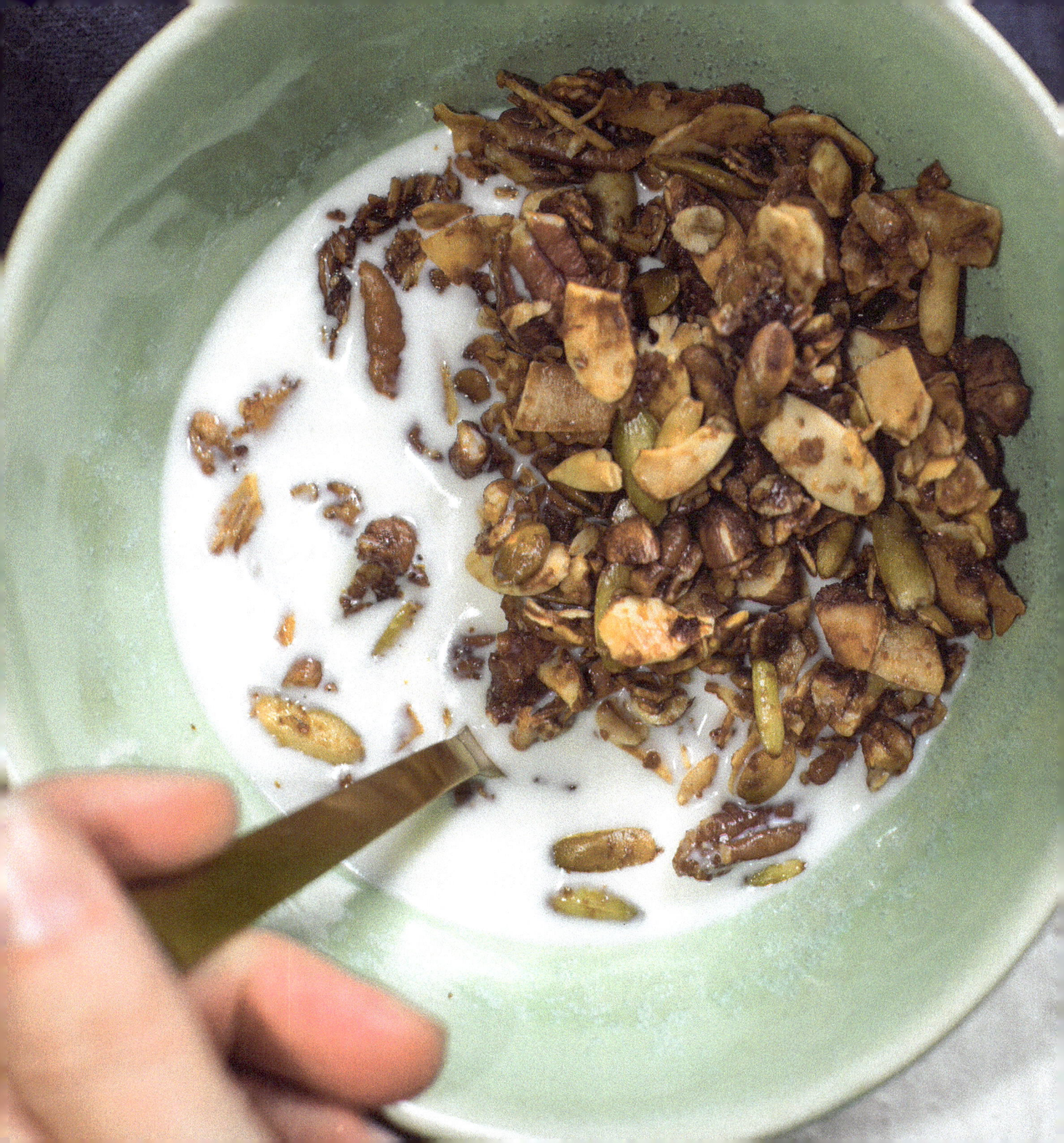

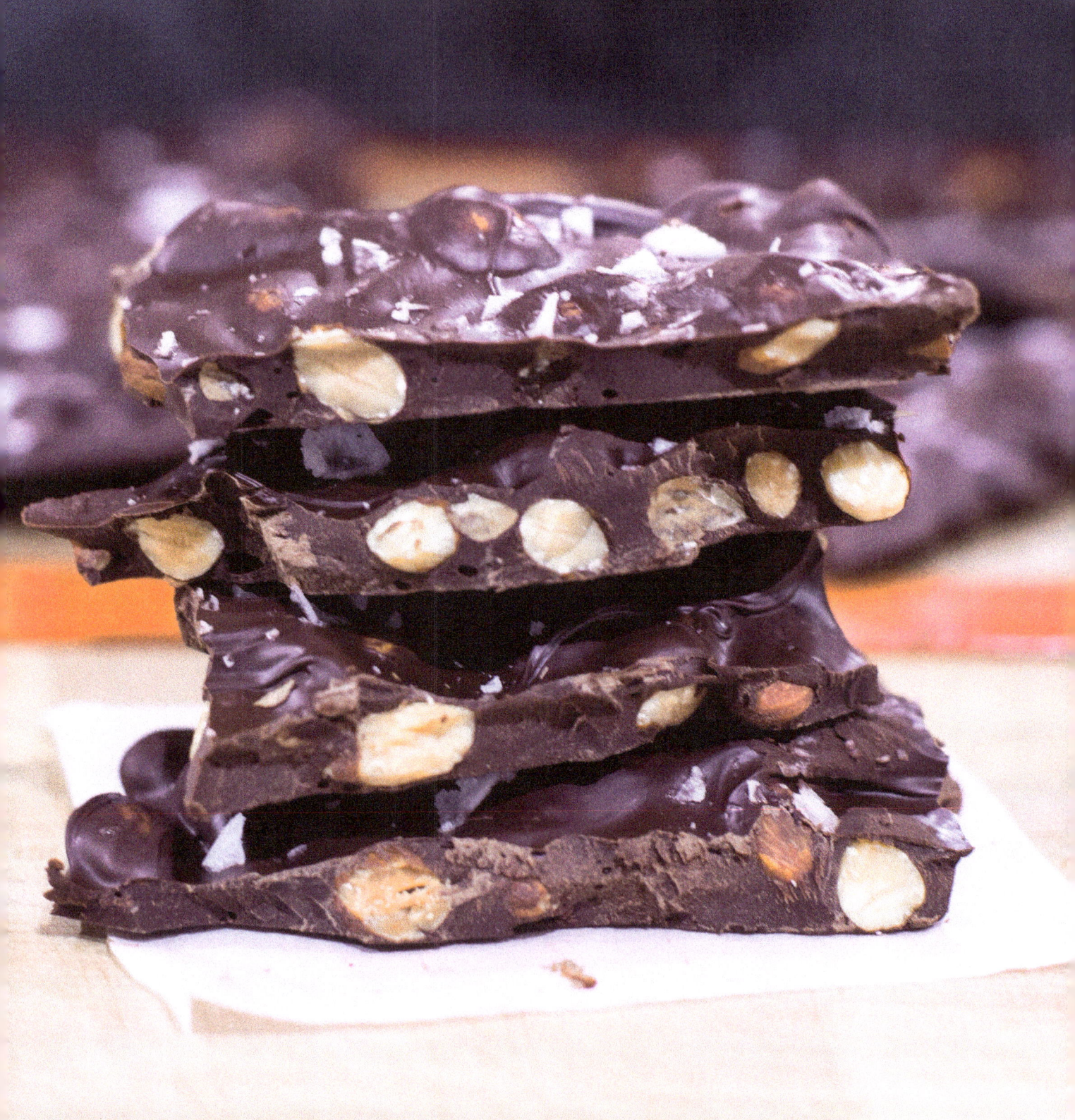

ALMOND BARK

MAKES 32 SERVINGS

Perfectly roasted almonds wrapped up in the richest, creamiest dark chocolate! Oh yeah — I'm in! This recipe is not only ridiculously easy, it's also so good. The only important thing to remember is that you need to use the most delicious chocolate you can find. Then use really good almonds. Using freshly roasted almonds will give you the best fresh roasty flavor. Adding a little fleur de sel or another craft salt to the top of this almond bark really takes it to the next level. All the flavors come together for a truly decadent snack. This stuff looks so fancy that I often give it out as gifts around the holidays.

INGREDIENTS

- 3 bags of high quality bittersweet chocolate chips, like Guittard brand
- 4 cups of roasted almonds, unsalted
- 1 tablespoon of Maldon salt OR other variety of craft salt.

DIRECTIONS

Place the chocolate chips in a microwave-safe bowl.

Microwave on high for 2 minutes. Stir.

Microwave for 2 more minutes. Stir.

Continue to microwave, 1 minute at a time, until the chocolate is completely melted.

Stir in the almonds.

Pour the mixture onto silpat or waxed paper.

Spread the mixture out to the thickness of about a finger's width.

Sprinkle with craft salt. I like pinot noir salt or salt crystals.

Place in the freezer until the bark is set.

Crack it apart into pieces.

Store in an airtight container. Store in the refrigerator if the weather is warm

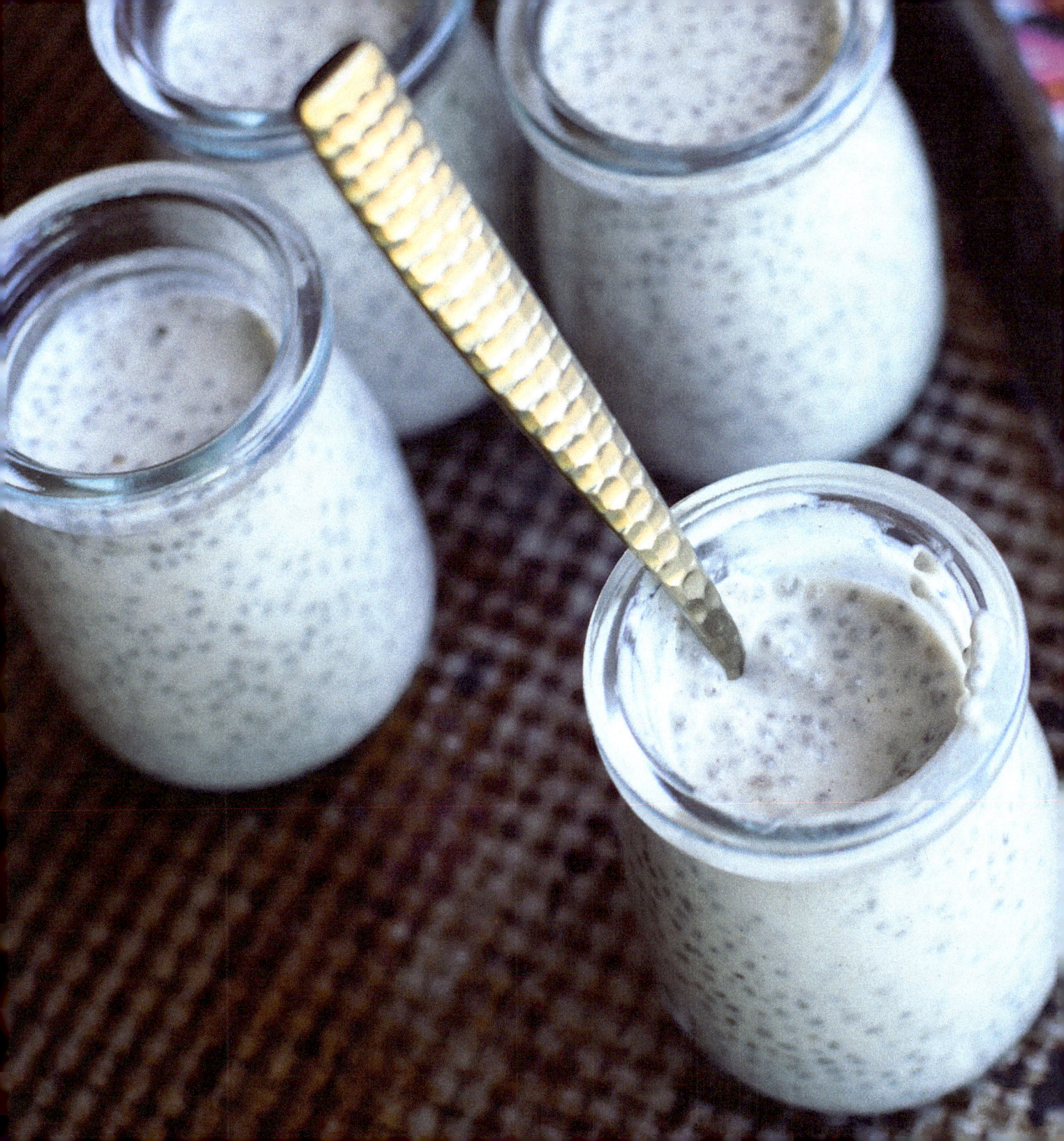

CHAI LATTE CHIA PUDDING

MAKES 12 SERVINGS

Imagine a rich, creamy chai latte in pudding form. It's smooth and spicy and packed with healthy coconut cream flavor. Eating it feels like cheating, but the nourishing collagen peptides packed into these little cups of deliciousness will give you a helping of gut-healing, protein building nourishment. These are pure guilt-free satisfaction.

INGREDIENTS

- 1 cup of extra strong chai tea
- 2 cans of coconut milk
- 2 tablespoons of raw honey, to taste
- 2 teaspoons of cinnamon
- ½ teaspoon of ground cardamom
- 1 teaspoon vanilla extract or 1 vanilla bean, scraped
- 4 scoops Vital Protein Collagen Peptides
- ½ cup chia seeds

DIRECTIONS

Brew a nice big cup of chai tea. To make this tea really strong, use 3 to 4 tea bags (or 3 to 4 teaspoons of loose tea) and 1 cup of water. Let the tea steep for about 5 minutes, and then squeeze the tea bags to get as much flavor as possible.

Whisk all the ingredients together.

Let sit for 10 minutes, then whisk again.

Pour into pudding cups or small ramekins.

Refrigerate for a few hours before serving. The pudding will thicken as it chills.

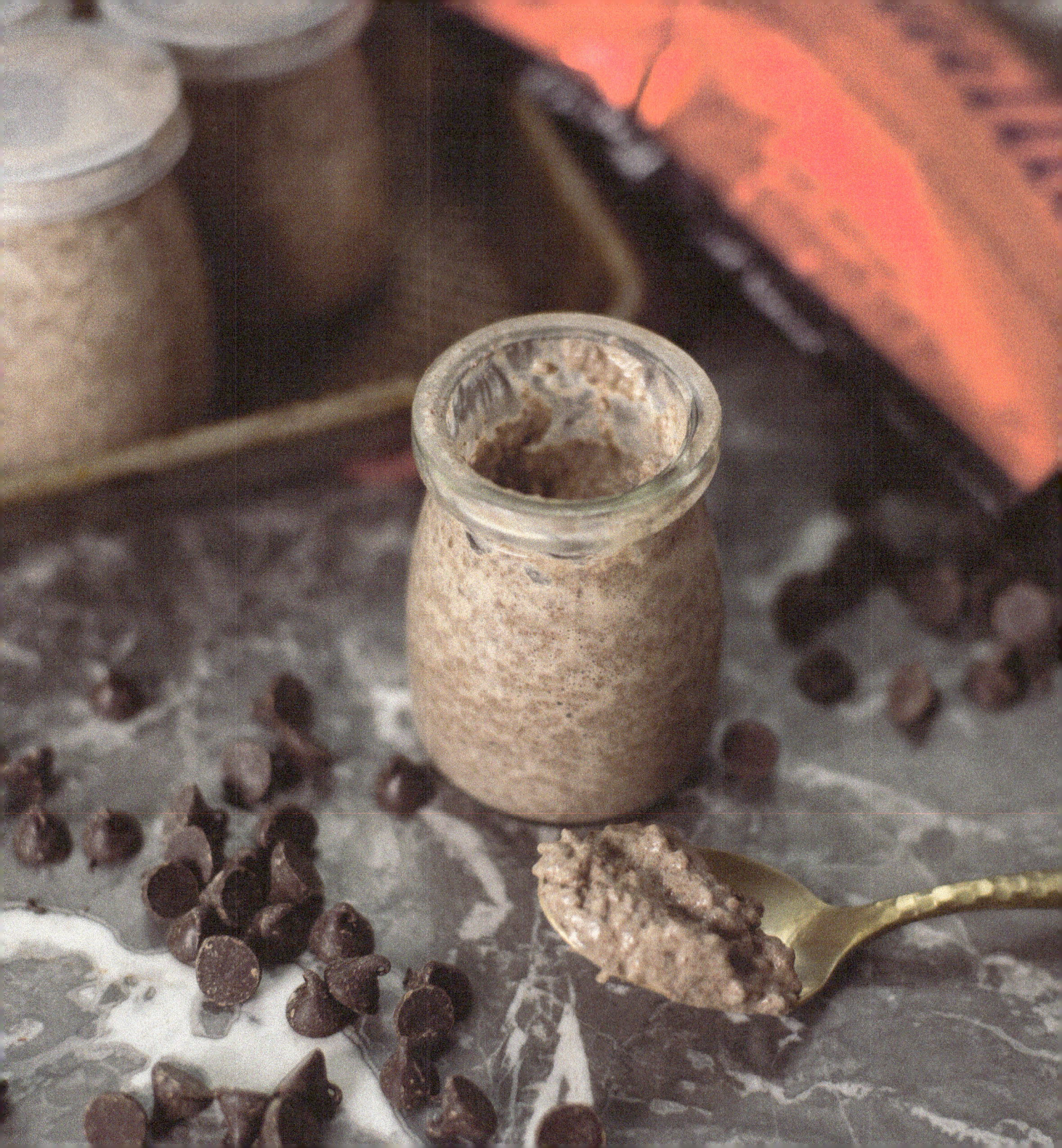

CHOCOLATE CHIA PUDDING

MAKES 12 SERVINGS

Creamy chocolate pudding cups? Sign me up! Who says you can't have your dessert and eat it, too? You'll feel good about indulging in a sweet treat that is lower in sugar, dairy-free, and full of healthy fats. Best of all, it only takes 5 minutes to make. If the mood strikes you, stir in a handful of mini marshmallows and crushed graham crackers at the very end to give it a S'mores vibe.

INGREDIENTS

⅔ cup chia seeds
2 cups full fat coconut milk
1 6.8-ounce container coconut cream
1 cup bittersweet chocolate chips
2 teaspoons vanilla
¼ teaspoon Kosher salt

PRO TIP: I use Kara brand coconut cream. You can find it stocked in many grocery stores in the ethnic aisle. It's packaged in a paper carton. If you can't find it at your local grocer, you can buy it online.

DIRECTIONS

Put the chia seeds in a large bowl. Set them aside.

Add the remaining ingredients to a high powered blender or food processor.

Blend until the chocolate is evenly incorporated.

Pour over chia seeds and whisk.

Let sit for 10 minutes.

Whisk again, then pour into 6 pudding cups or small ramekins.

Refrigerate for a few hours before serving. The pudding will thicken as it chills.

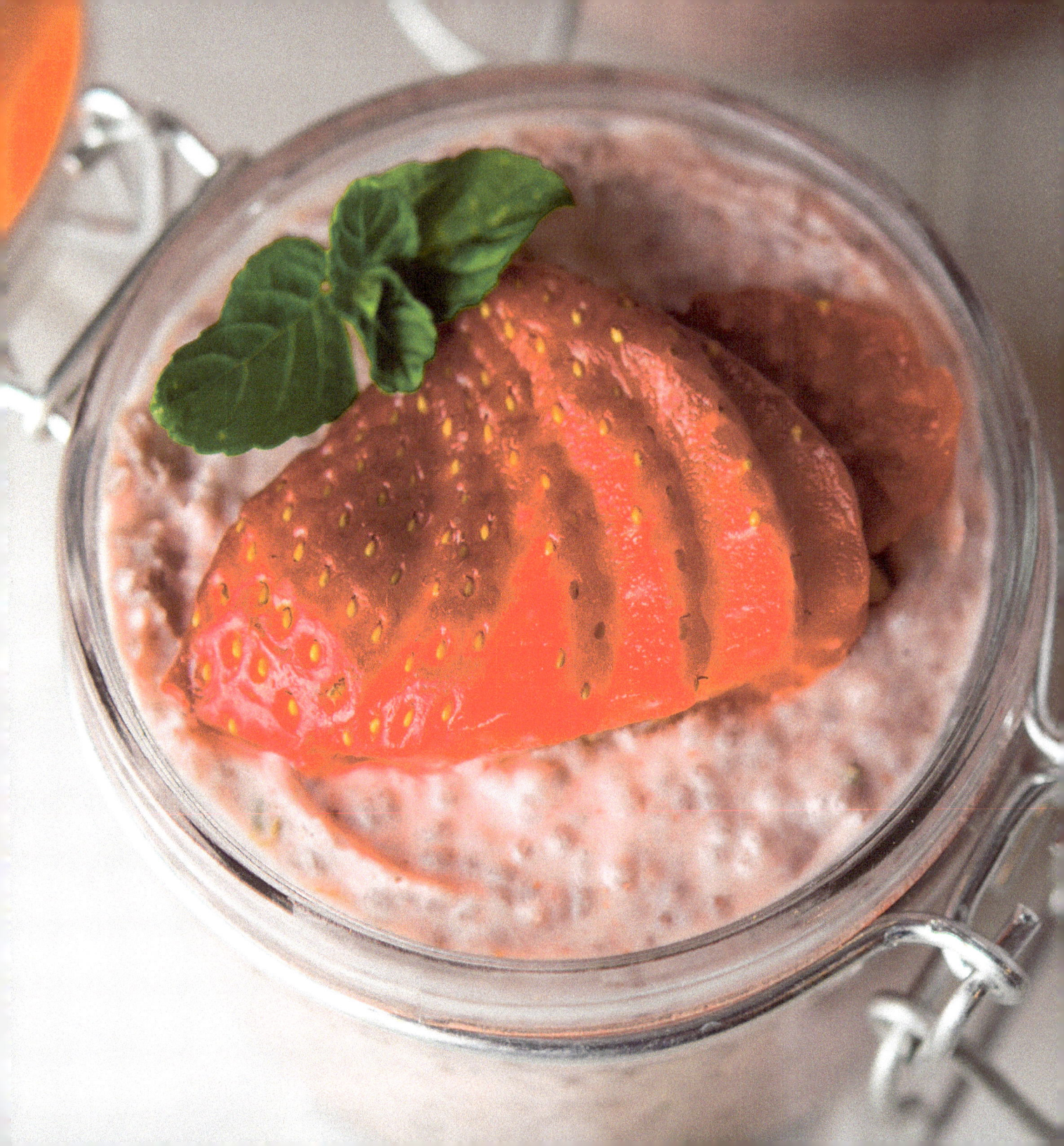

STRAWBERRY CHIA PUDDING

MAKES 12 SERVINGS

This strawberry pudding tastes like fresh strawberries and cream. It's not only a dairy-free treat, but it's also a full serving of Omega-3s. This recipe is really flexible; you can swap the strawberries out with any fruit that you like. I especially love a tropical spin with mangoes and shredded coconut.

INGREDIENTS

- ⅔ to ¾ cup chia seeds
- 2 ½ cups fresh strawberries
- 1 13.5-ounce can full-fat coconut milk
- 1 6.8-ounce container coconut cream, like Kara brand
- 1 lime, zested
- ½ lime, juiced
- 1 vanilla bean, scraped
- ¼ cup honey or agave

DIRECTIONS

Place the chia seeds in a large bowl and set them aside.

Add the remaining ingredients to a high powered blender or food processor. Puree until smooth.

Pour the pureed mixture over the chia seeds and whisk.

Let set for 10 minutes.

Whisk again and then pour into 6 pudding cups or small ramekins.

Refrigerate for a few hours before serving. The pudding will thicken as it chills.

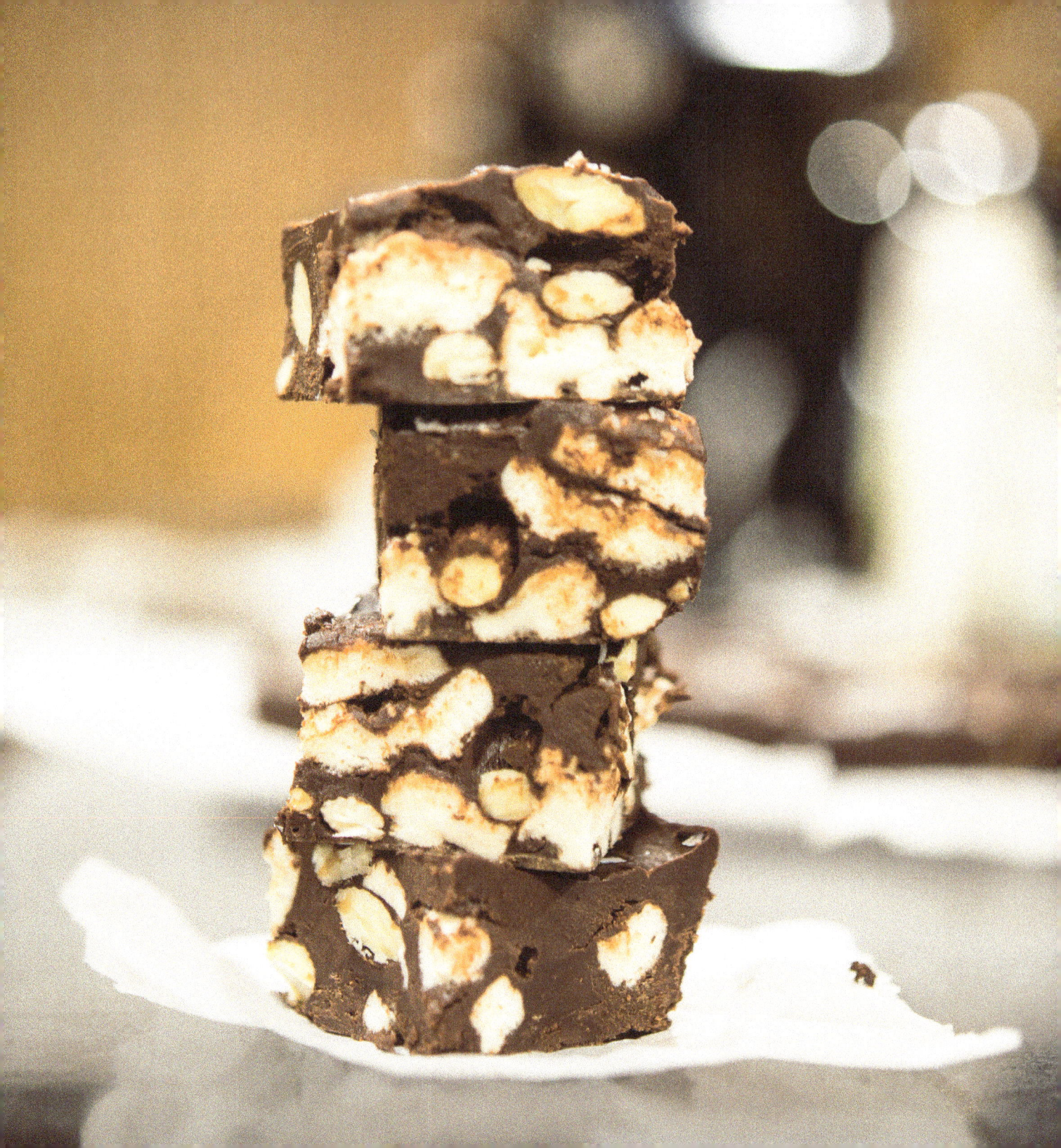

ROCKY ROAD FUDGE

MAKES 16 SERVINGS

Crunchy, toasted almonds and soft, fluffy marshmallows swimming in dark chocolate. This stuff is a candy bar-status confection! Using dark chocolate makes this sweet treat naturally dairy-free. This is another 5-minute prep time dessert. It can be our little secret that you make it in the microwave!

Absolutely any type of dried fruit and nuts can be mixed into the melted chocolate, and you could easily make this fudge without the nuts and marshmallows. Go wild and experiment with adding your favorite mix-ins!

INGREDIENTS

- 16 ounces chocolate chips
- 1 cup coconut cream
- 1 cup mini marshmallows
- 1 cup roasted almonds, whole or roughly chopped
- Sprinkle of flake salt (optional, but worth it!)

DIRECTIONS

Microwave the chocolate chips for 1 minute on high, then stir. Repeat up to 3 times or until the chocolate is melted and smooth.

Add the coconut cream and stir until well blended.

Add the nuts and marshmallows.

Pour into a square silicone baking pan or a pan lined with foil or parchment.

Place in the freezer until the fudge is set.

Sprinkle with flake salt.

Cut into bite-sized pieces.

NOTES

VEGAN ADAPTABLE: Use vegan marshmallows, like Dandies brand. Dark chocolate is usually dairy-free.

ALTERNATIVE MIX-INS: mini peanut butter cups, Reese's Pieces, shredded coconut, walnuts or cashews, dried cranberries... There are so many options here.

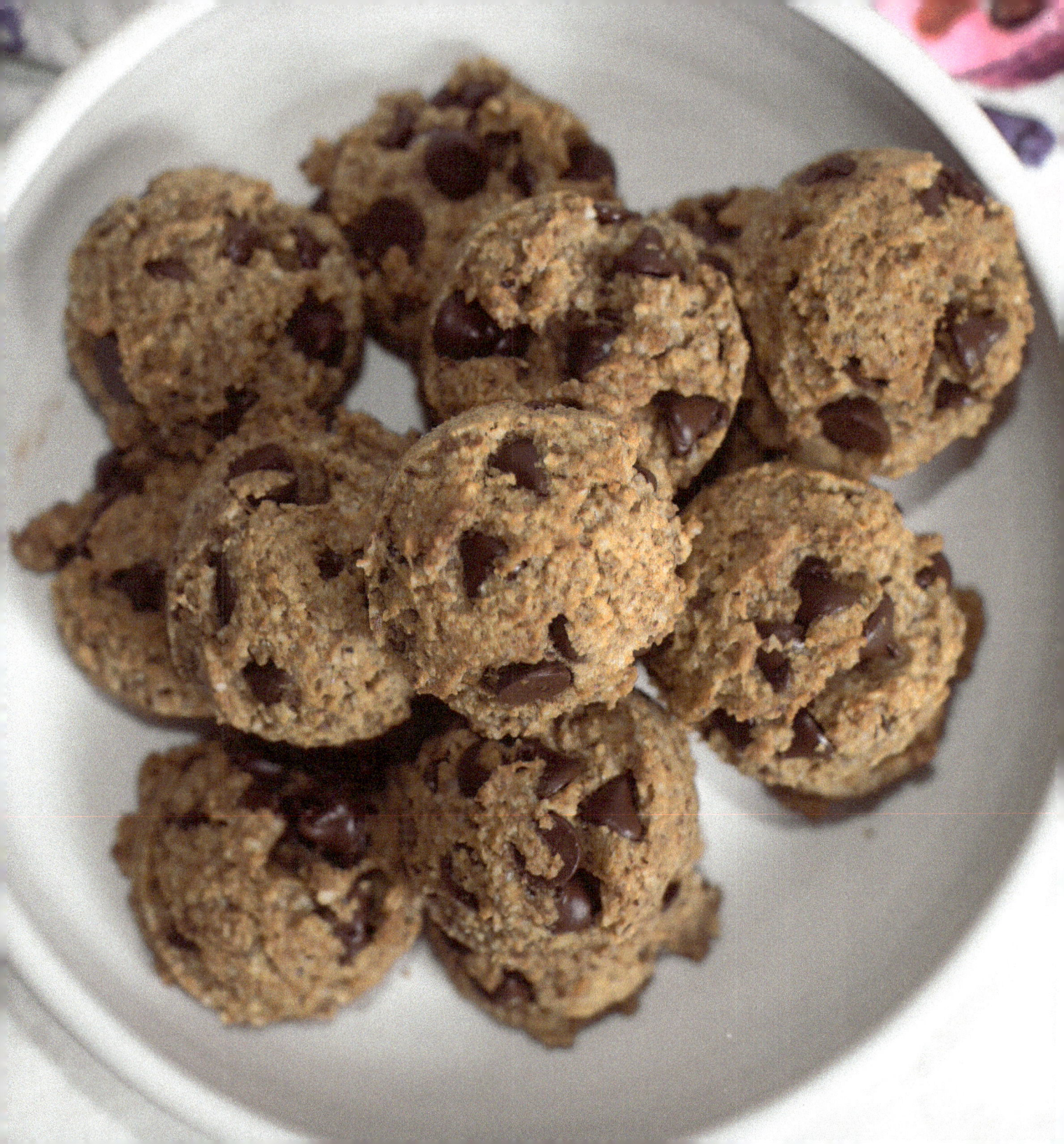

HAZELNUT CHOCOLATE CHIP COOKIES

MAKES 24 COOKIES

Chocolate chip cookies are life. If you've been avoiding gluten and haven't been able to have chocolate chip cookies, fear not! The hazelnut flour bakes into a perfect texture and has a rich, roasted, gourmet flavor. So go ahead, kill that chocolate chip cookie craving.

INGREDIENTS

- 3 cups hazelnut flour or meal
- 1 teaspoon baking soda
- 1 teaspoon Kosher salt
- ½ cup coconut oil, melted
- ½ cup maple syrup
- 2 eggs
- 1 teaspoon vanilla
- 1 ½ cups chocolate chips

DIRECTIONS

Preheat the oven to 375°F.

Combine the dry ingredients in a medium bowl.

In a second bowl, beat the wet ingredients with a hand mixer until combined.

Pour the wet ingredients into the dry ingredients and beat until combined.

Stir in the chocolate chips.

Drop balls of cookie dough (about 1 tablespoon in size) onto a parchment-lined baking sheet.

Bake for 10 to 12 minutes until the cookies are just browned on the edges. Cool before serving.

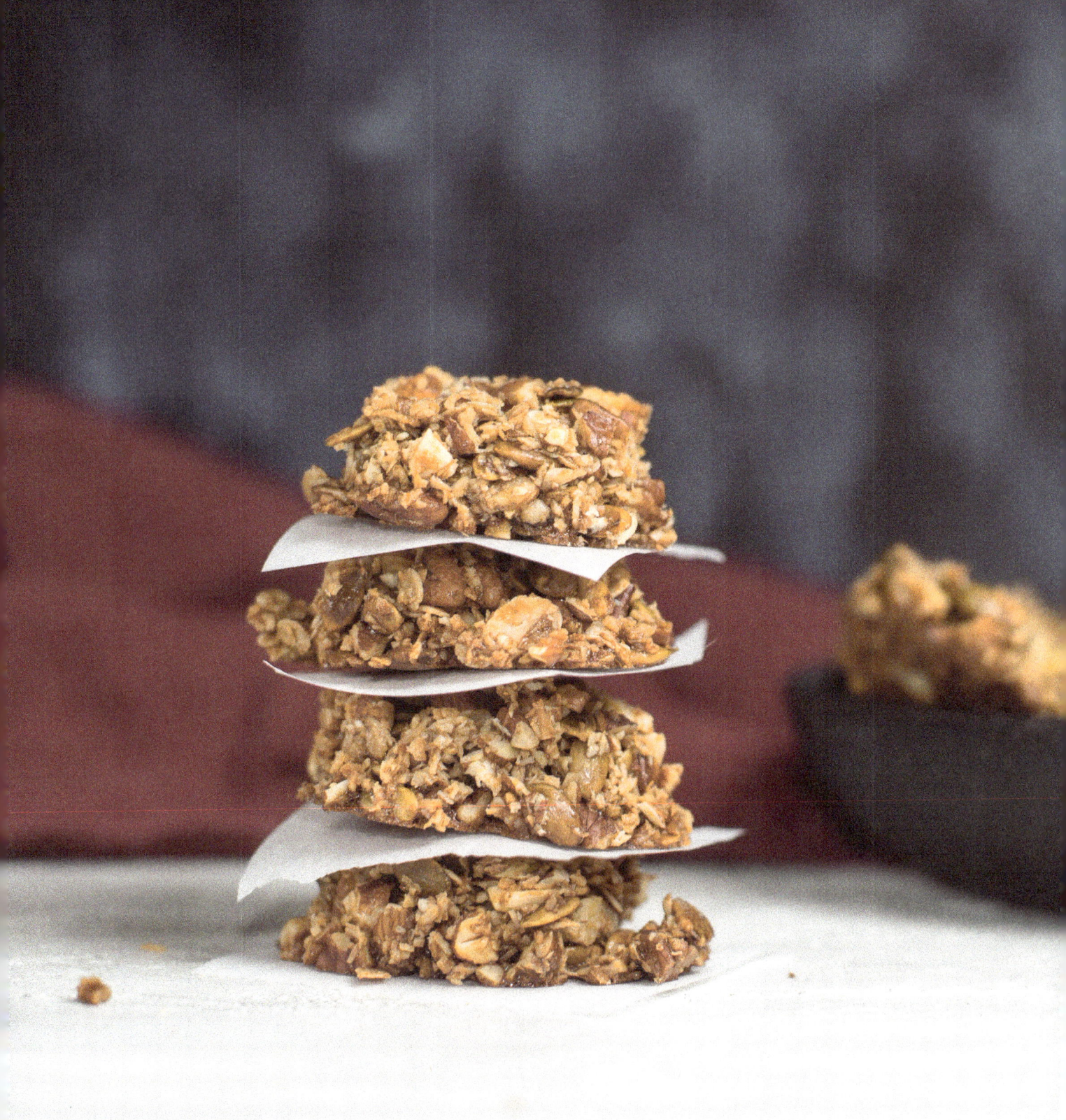

PALEO GRANOLA BITES

MAKES 72 COOKIES

Imagine the best granola you've ever had, in cookie form. Or if you would rather make this mixture up as a batch of granola, just spread it out on a baking sheet lined with parchment paper. Bake until it is nice and toasty and serve with almond milk and a big spoon! Either way, this will be one of those recipes that you'll make over and over again.

INGREDIENTS

- 3 cups pecan pieces
- 2 cups almonds, sliced
- 2 cups unsweetened coconut, shredded or flaked
- 1½ cups pepitas (pumpkin seeds), shelled
- 1 cup oats
- 1 teaspoon Kosher salt
- 6 tablespoons coconut oil, melted
- 4 egg whites, whisked
- 1⅓ cups coconut sugar

DIRECTIONS

Preheat the oven to 325°F.

Mix the dry ingredients and coconut oil in a large bowl, and then spread the mixture on a rimmed baking sheet.

Bake 10 minutes, then let it cool.

Whisk the egg whites in a large bowl until they are foamy. Gradually add the coconut sugar while continuing to whisk.

Add the wet and dry mixtures together. (It doesn't matter which you add to the other.) Stir until well incorporated.

Use a tablespoon or a cookie scoop to drop spoonfuls of the mixture onto a parchment-lined baking sheet. Space them evenly. You can place your cookies pretty close to one another. They will not spread much.

Bake 15 to 20 minutes until the cookies are golden brown. Transfer them to a wire rack to cool. (They will get crispier as they cool.)

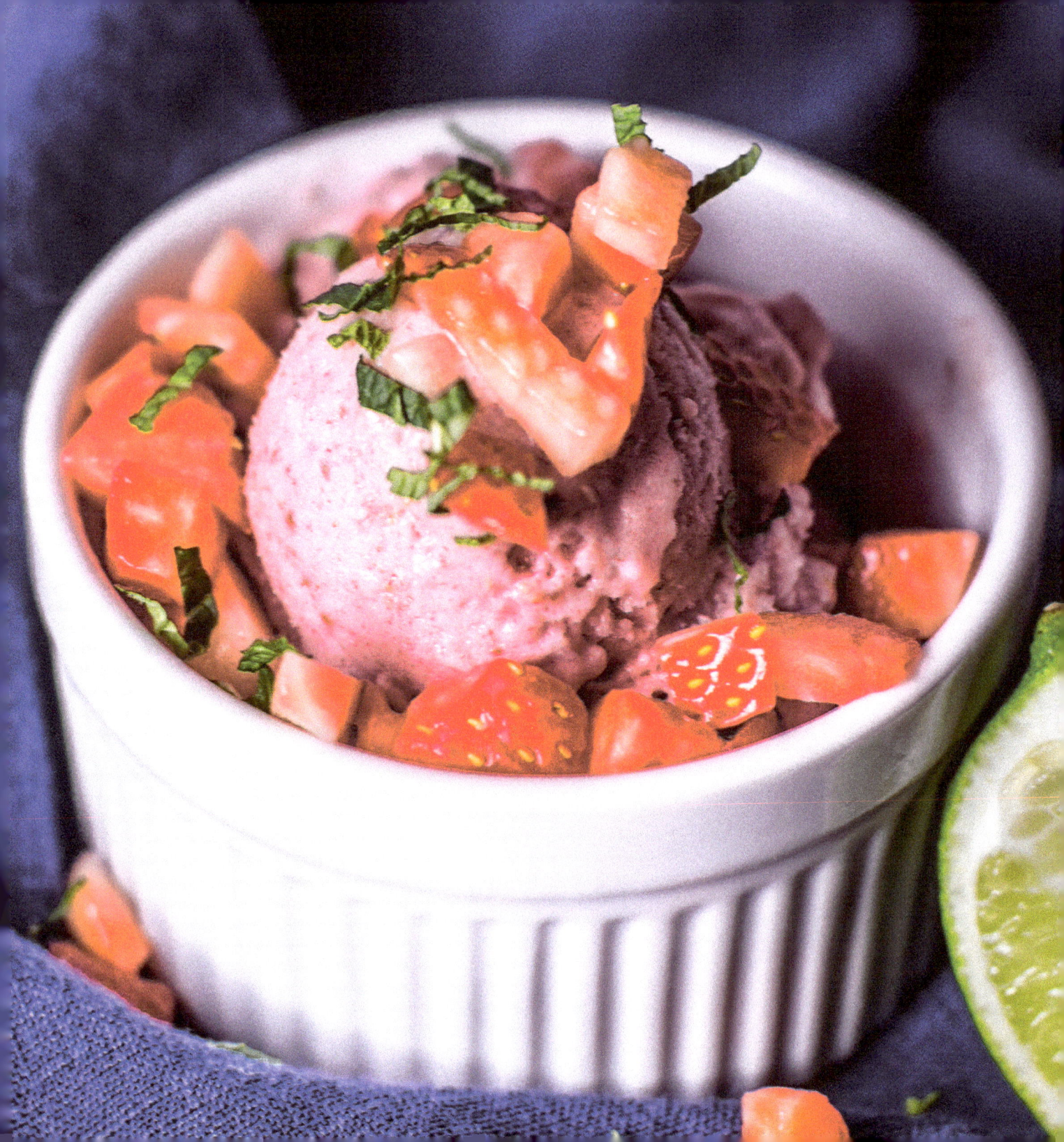

STRAWBERRY MOJITO NICE CREAM

MAKES 6 TO 8 SERVINGS

What is Nice Cream, you ask? Nice Cream is a dairy-free version of ice cream that is sweetened with fruit instead of processed sugar. When you're craving the sweet, cold creaminess of ice cream but don't want all the processed ingredients, Nice Cream is the perfect solution. You can make it a million different ways, but this Strawberry Mojito version is one of my favorites.

INGREDIENTS

6 frozen bananas
2 cups frozen strawberries
4 ounces coconut cream
1 lime, juiced
1 teaspoon fresh mint
Fresh strawberries, chopped
Fresh mint, chopped
Lime, a fresh squeeze on top

DIRECTIONS

Add all the ingredients to a high powered blender.

Blend until creamy.

NOTE

You can eat this Nice Cream right out of the blender (it may be on the softer side), or you can put it in an airtight container and freeze it. For future snacking, set it out for about 5 to 10 minutes before scooping.

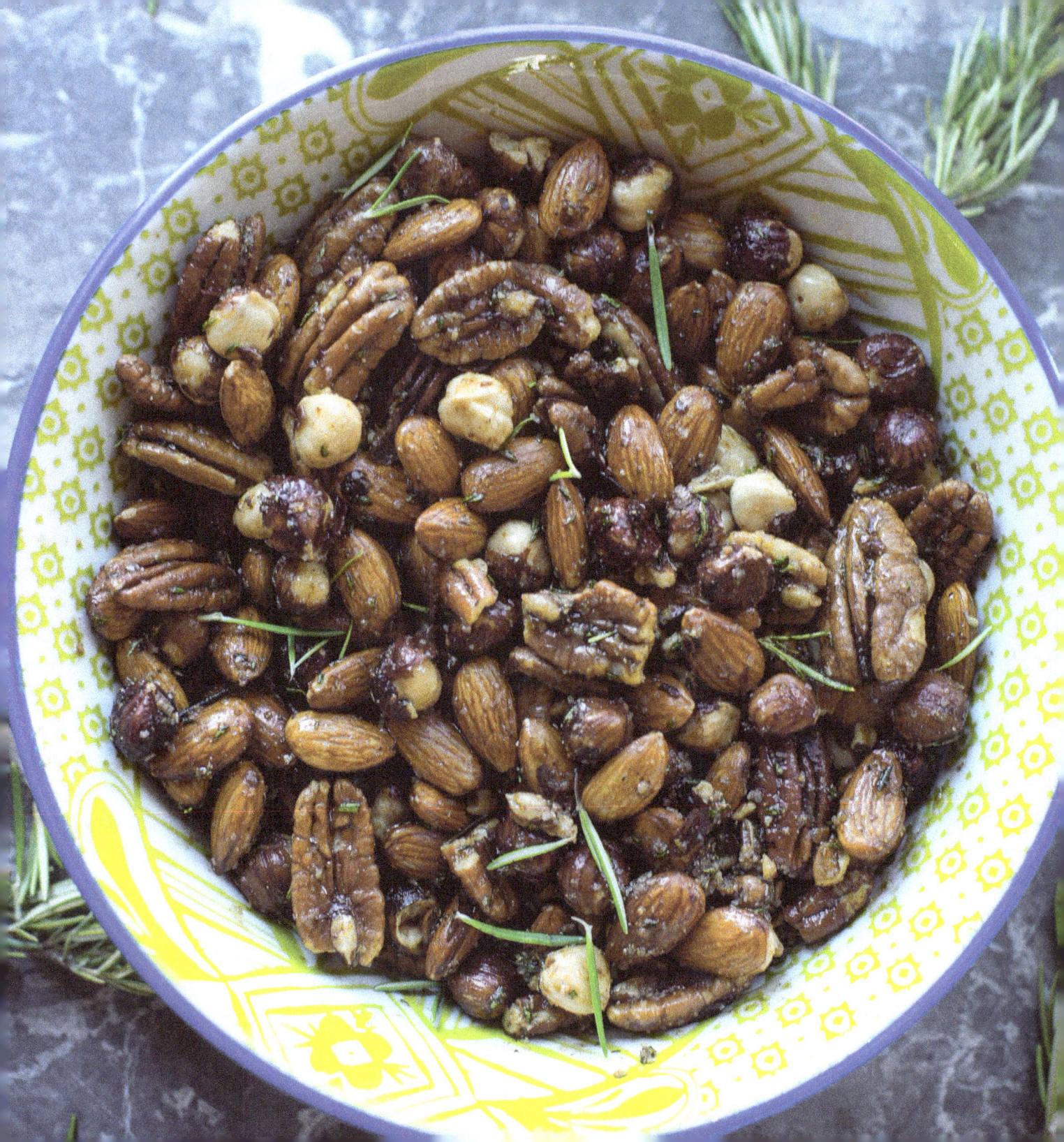

SAVORY ROASTED NUTS

MAKES 24 SERVINGS

When it comes to snacking, nuts are it! Toasty roasted nuts with a little salt and a lotta spice are my favorite crunchtastic go-to snack. Because they're ultra-portable, they are perfect for curbing hunger any time, anywhere.

INGREDIENTS

- 1 pound nuts (try almonds, pecans, and hazelnuts)
- ¼ cup avocado oil
- 1 tablespoon fresh rosemary, chopped
- ½ tablespoon coarse salt
- ½ teaspoon chili powder
- ½ teaspoon paprika
- ½ teaspoon cayenne
- ½ teaspoon dry mustard powder
- ½ teaspoon garlic powder
- ¼ teaspoon cinnamon
- ⅛ teaspoon nutmeg
- ⅛ teaspoon allspice

DIRECTIONS

Preheat the oven to 325°F.

Roast the nuts on a baking sheet for about 15 minutes. Watch them closely so that they do not burn.

Heat the avocado oil and spices in a heavy skillet.

Add the warm nuts to the warmed spices and toss well.

Spread the nuts on a baking sheet and let them cool.

Store in an airtight container.

APPENDIX
WHAT TO MAKE TONIGHT?

Best Laid Plans

Be flexible! Even if one Beast Bowl recipe is built with chicken, you can always swap the poultry out for a different core protein. I have tried to provide suggestions for each recipe. There are also many options for making every Beast Bowl entirely plant-based.

Planning takes a little practice. Start slowly by picking 1 or 2 core proteins for the week. Then add a few Extras. I have a ton of helpful planning sheets on the blog to get you started. I've found that different systems work for different people. Experimenting will help you figure out what works for you.

My *Pick 2* downloads will help to get you started. Each one contains a grocery list and an action plan that will take the guesswork out of meal prep this week.

You can always find me at FoodologyGeek.com/BBN I hope to see you there!

GOT CHICKEN?

Asian Chicken Meatballs /47
Buffalo Style Chicken /87
Pulled *Chicken* Barbecue /79
Chicken Chile Verde /65
Chicken Lettuce Wraps /133
Chicken Satay /61
Chipotle Chicken /69
Fried Chicken /83
Greek *Chicken* Burger /115
Provençel Chicken /103
Jamaican Jerk Chicken /107
Lemongrass *Chicken* /53
Mediterranean *Chicken* /123
Chicken Chimichurri /93
Chicken Taco /99
Chicken Teriyaki /57
Tequila Lime *Chicken* /75

GOT BEEF?

All-American Burger /89
Beef Teriyaki /57
Chipotle *Beef* /69
Mom-Style Taco /99
Greek *Beef* Burger /115
Steak & Sweet Potato /127
Steak Chimichurri /93

GOT PORK?

Asian *Pork* Meatballs /47
Barbecue Pulled Pork /79
Chipotle *Pork*/69
Lemongrass *Pork* /53
Pork Chile Verde /65

GOT SEAFOOD?

Buffalo Style *Shrimp* /87
Chipotle *Shrimp*/69
Shrimp Chimichurri /93
Lemongrass Shrimp /53
Mediterranean *Shrimp* /123
Shrimp Teriyaki /57
Tequila Lime *Shrimp* /75

CORE PROTEINS

All-American Burger /89
Amped Up Scrambled Eggs /43
Asian Chicken Meatballs /47
Barbecue Pulled Pork /79
Buffalo Chicken /87
Chicken Chili Verde /65
Chicken Lettuce Wraps /133
Chicken Satay /61
Chipotle Chicken /69
Colombian Hanger Steak /93
Fried Chicken /83
Greek Lamb Burger /115
Jerk Chicken /107
Lemongrass Shrimp /53
Mediterranean Fish /123
Mom-Style Taco /99
Provençal Chicken /103
Shrimp Louie /125
Steak /127
Teriyaki /57
Tequila Lime Fish /75

PLANT-BASED

All-American Burger /89
Asian Meatballs /47
Barbecue *Jackfruit* /79
Breakfast Hash /45
Lettuce Wraps /133
Veggie Satay /61
Vegetarian Chili Verde /65
Cauliflower Chimichurri /93
Chipotle *Veggies* /69
Greek *Roasted Veggies* /115
Provençel *Roasted Veggies* /103
Jamaican Jerk *Mushrooms* /107
Lemongrass *Tofu* /53
Mediterranean *Tofu* /123
Vegetarian Mom-Style Taco /99
Mushroom & Sweet Potato /127
Paleo Breakfast /43
Mushroom Teriyaki /57
Tequila Lime *Tofu and Chickpeas*/75

Acknowledgements

There is not enough space here to express the gratitude that I have for all the people in my life that have helped me get to this place.

To my husband Brad, your unwavering support and belief in me, as well as your continuous encouragement, help me to get past my inner mean girl. Thank you for being my ride or die.

To my parents, who gave me what I needed to be a fighter, your guidance has made me self-reliant and a relentless pursuer of being better every single day.

To my Aunt Sheila, you have always loved me without judgement or question. You've been there in my life to remind me and encourage me through every mistake and every wrong decision and to cheer me on when I felt lost. You helped me to be kinder to myself. Thank you for your constant love and support.

To Karie, I am so grateful that you came into my life. Your editing chops really made this cookbook better than it could have ever been without you. Thank you so much for your excitement about this project and your dedication to making this cookbook super rad!

To Kit, your encouragement and belief in Foodology Geek allowed me to reach for something bigger. Thank you for being there and helping me get this thing rolling. Here's to all the cake and whiskey days.

Tiffany, your advice and inspiration have helped me in countless ways in so many areas of my life. Thank you for being in my life through thick and thin.

To Cassandra, you are a complete rock star. Thank you so much for the push I needed to to step off the cliff into the abyss of this thing called entrepreneurship. You're a queen, and you always inspire me to keep reaching. We got this, sister!

To my cheerleaders, Jessica, Lisa, Nancy, Barbara, and Katy. Thank you for the encouragement when I felt like giving up and all of the inspiration that keeps me focused on building this crazy dream! We can all do this!

To all of my family and friends along the way that have encouraged and believed in me, I'm grateful for all of you. I'm so fortunate to be surrounded by many strong, beautiful people that believe in building one another up!

INDEX

A

All-American Burger 89
Almond Bark 193
almonds 33
    Almond Bark 193
    Rocky Road Fudge 201
apple cider vinegar 80
apples
    Carrot & Apple Slaw 135
aromatics 7
Asian Chicken Meatball 47
Asian Cucumber Salad 49
Asian Dressing 49
Asian Peanut Dressing 51
Asian Slaw 51
avocado mayonnaise 80
avocado oil 9
avocados
    Columbian Guacamole 97
    Mexican Guacamole 67

B

bacon
    Fried Chicken 83
balsamic vinegar
    Tomato Balsamic Vinaigrette 147
barbecue
    Barbecue Pulled Pork 79
    Peach Bourbon Barbecue Sauce 175
    Spicy Tangy Barbecue Sauce 173
Barbecue Pulled Pork 79
basic kitchen tools 63
Beastastic Mayo 153
Beast Bowls
    All-American Burger 89
    Asian Chicken Meatball 47
    Barbecue Pulled Pork 79
    Buffalo Chicken 87
    Chicken Satay 61
    Chili Verde 65
    Chipotle Chicken 69
    Fried Chicken 83
    Greek Lamb Burger 115
    Jamaican Jerk Chicken 107
    Lemongrass Shrimp 53
    Mediterranean 123
    Mom-Style Taco 99
    Paleo Breakfast 43
    Provençal Chicken & Veggies 103
    Shrimp Louie 125
    Steak & Sweet Potato 127
    Tequila Lime Fish 75
Beast Sauce 158
beef
    All-American Burger 89
    Greek Lamb Burger 115
    Mom-Style Taco 99
    Paleo Meatloaf 119
    Steak Chimichurri 93
    Steak & Sweet Potato 127
Blanched Green Beans 105, 121
blueberries
    Paleo Breakfast 43
bone broth 33
breakfast
    Breakfast Hash 45
    Paleo Breakfast 43
Breakfast Hash 45
brown mustard
    Mustard Vinaigrette 145
Buffalo Chicken 87
Buffalo Ranch 156
Buttermilk Marinade 83

C

cabbage
    Asian Slaw 51
    Mexican Slaw 101
    Southern Coleslaw 80
carbohydrates 10
Carrot & Apple Slaw 135
carrots
    Carrot & Apple Slaw 135
    Mexican Slaw 101
    Southern Coleslaw 80
cauliflower
    Cauliflower Smash 121
Cauliflower Smash 121
celery salt 80
celery seed 80
chai latte
    Chai Latte Chia Pudding 195
Chai Latte Chia Pudding 195
chai tea
    Chai Latte Chia Pudding 195
Champagne Vinaigrette 142
champagne vinegar
    Champagne Vinaigrette 142
    Citrus Vinaigrette 142
    Herbes de Provence Vinaigrette 144
chia seeds
    Chai Latte Chia Pudding 195
    Chocolate Chia Pudding 197
    Strawberry Chia Pudding 199
chicken
    Asian Chicken Meatball 47
    Buffalo Chicken 87
    Chicken Lettuce Wraps 133
    Chicken Satay 61
    Chili Verde 65
    Chipotle Chicken 69
    Fried Chicken 83
    Jamaican Jerk Chicken 107
    Provençal Chicken & Veggies 103
    Teriyaki Chicken 57
Chicken Lettuce Wraps 133
Chicken Satay 61
Chili Verde 65

Chimichurri Sauce 165
Chipotle Chicken 69
Chipotle Ranch 157
chocolate
    Almond Bark 193
    Chocolate Chia Pudding 197
    Rocky Road Fudge 201
Chocolate Chia Pudding 197
chocolate chips
    Hazelnut Chocolate Chip Cookies 203
choosing fish 76
cinnamon
    Chai Latte Chia Pudding 195
Citrus Vinaigrette 142
coconut cream
    Chocolate Chia Pudding 197
    Rocky Road Fudge 201
    Strawberry Mojito Nice Cream 207
coconut milk
    Chai Latte Chia Pudding 195
    Paleo Ranch 155
    Strawberry Chia Pudding 199
coconut oil 19
coleslaw
    Southern Coleslaw 80
Coleslaw Dressing 80
collagen peptides
    Chai Latte Chia Pudding 195
Columbian Guacamole 97
condiment
    Onion Jam 177
    Paleo Ketchup 167
    Spicy Tomato Jam 179
cookies
    Hazelnut Chocolate Chip Cookies 203
core protein 21
corn
    Roasted Corn Salsa 71
cucumber
    Asian Cucumber Salad 49

D

daikon 55
dairy free
    Chai Latte Chia Pudding 195
    Chocolate Chia Pudding 197
    Strawberry Chia Pudding 199
dietary fat 9
dijon mustard
    Tomato Balsamic Vinaigrette 147
dressing
    Asian Dressing 49
    Asian Peanut Slaw Dressing 51
    Beastastic Mayo 153
    Beast Sauce 158
    Buffalo Ranch 156
    Champagne Vinaigrette 142
    Chipotle Ranch 157
    Citrus Vinaigrette 142
    Coleslaw Dressing 80
    Greek Vinaigrette 144
    Herbes de Provence Vinaigrette 144
    Lemon Tahini Dressing 171
    Louie Dressing 125, 158
    Mustard Vinaigrette 145
    Paleo Ranch 155
    Red Wine Vinaigrette 145
    Satay Peanut Sauce 181
    Sesame Ginger Vinaigrette 147
    Tomato Balsamic Vinaigrette 147

E

eggs
    Breakfast Hash 45
    Paleo Breakfast 43
extras 6

F

fasting 13
feta
    Greek Vinaigrette 144
fish
    choosing fish 76
    Mediterranean 123
    Tequila Lime Fish 75
fish sauce 53
fixins 6
Fried Chicken 83
fries
    Sweet Potato Fries 131
frozen meats 36
fudge
    Rocky Road Fudge 201
furikake 57

G

garlic
    Sesame Ginger Vinaigrette 147
ginger 53
    Sesame Ginger Vinaigrette 147
gluten free
    Fried Chicken 83
granola
    Paleo Granola Bites 205
grass-fed 37
Greek
    Tzatziki 169
Greek Lamb Burger 115
Greek Vinaigrette 144
green beans
    Blanched Green Beans 105, 121
guacamole
    Columbian Guacamole 97
    Mexican Guacamole 67
gut health 12

H

Hazelnut Chocolate Chip Cookies 203
hazelnut flour
   Hazelnut Chocolate Chip Cookies 203
healthy fats 9
herbes de provence
   Herbes de Provence Vinaigrette 144
Herbes de Provence Vinaigrette 144
honey
   Chai Latte Chia Pudding 195
   Strawberry Chia Pudding 199
How To Meal Prep 59, 63, 85
hunger 28

I

IF 13
insulin 8
insulin resistant 9
insulin spike 8

J

jam
   Onion Jam 177
   Spicy Tomato Jam 179
Jamaican Jerk Chicken 107
Jamaican Rice & Peas 113

K

kale 7
keto 11
ketogenic 10
kimchi 57

L

lamb
   Greek Lamb Burger 115
lean protein 8
leftover chicken 33
lemon
   Greek Vinaigrette 144
lemongrass 53
   Lemongrass Shrimp 53
   Lemongrass Marinade 53
Lemongrass Shrimp 53
Lemon Tahini Dressing 171
lettuces 7
lettuce wraps
   Barbecue Pulled Pork 79
   Chicken Lettuce Wraps 133
limes
   Strawberry Mojito Nice Cream 207
lose body fat 8
Louie Dressing 125, 158
low carb 10
luxury kitchen tools 85

M

macronutrients 5
mangoes
   Mango Salsa 77
Mango Salsa 77
maple syrup
   Hazelnut Chocolate Chip Cookies 203
marinades
   Buttermilk Marinade 83
   Lemongrass Marinade 53
   Satay Marinade 61
   Tequila Lime Marinade 75
   Teriyaki Marinade 57
marshmallows
   Rocky Road Fudge 201

N

mashed cauliflower
   Cauliflower Smash 121
mayo 148
   Beastastic Mayo 153
mayonnaise 148
meal prep 35
meatloaf
   Paleo Meatloaf 119
Mediterranean 123
metabolism 7
Mexican Guacamole 67
Mexican Slaw 101
microgreens 7, See also sprouts
micro-nutrition 5
mojito
   Strawberry Mojito Nice Cream 207
Mom-Style Taco 99
muscle growth 9
mustard
   Mustard Vinaigrette 145
Mustard Vinaigrette 145

N

nice cream
   Strawberry Mojito Nice Cream 207
non-dairy options 121
nuts, See also seeds
   Paleo Granola Bites 205
   Savory Roasted Nuts 209

O

oats
   Paleo Granola Bites 205
olive oil 9
onion
   Onion Jam 177
orange juice
   Citrus Vinaigrette 142
oregano

Greek Vinaigrette 144
Oven Roasted Potatoes 129

P

Paleo Breakfast 43
Paleo Granola Bites 205
Paleo Ketchup 167
Paleo Meatloaf 119
Paleo Ranch 155
panchetta
   Breakfast Hash 45
Peach Bourbon Barbecue Sauce 175
peanut
   Asian Peanut Dressing 51
peanuts
   Satay Peanut Sauce 181
pecans
   Paleo Granola Bites 205
phytonutrients 7
pickled
   Pickled Asian Veggies 55
Pickled Asian Veggies 55
pick two 33
pineapple
   Pineapple Salsa 110
Pineapple Salsa 110
plantains
   Roasted Plantains 109
   Tostones 95
pork
   Barbecue Pulled Pork 79
   Breakfast Hash 45
pork shoulder 79
portion control 27
portion control guidelines 28
   female 28
   male 29
potatoes
   Oven Roasted Potatoes 129
   Sweet Potato Fries 131
prep 34

protein
   must-have proteins 37
Provençal Chicken & Veggies 103
pudding
   Chai Latte Chia Pudding 195
   Strawberry Chia Pudding 199

R

red beans
   Jamaican Rice & Peas 113
Red Wine Vinaigrette 145
red wine vinegar
   Greek Vinaigrette 144
   Red Wine Vinaigrette 145
Remoulade 159
rice
   Chili Verde 65
   Jamaican Rice & Peas 113
   Teriyaki Chicken 57
rice wine vinegar 55
   Sesame Ginger Vinaigrette 147
Roasted Corn Salsa 71
roasted garlic 121
Roasted Plantains 109
Rocky Road Fudge 201
rosemary
   Savory Roasted Nuts 209

S

salsa
   Mango Salsa 77
   Pineapple Salsa 110
   Salsa Fresca 72
Salsa Fresca 72
Satay Marinade 61
Satay Peanut Sauce 181
satiety cues 28, 30
sauce
   Beastastic Mayo 153

Beast Sauce 158
Chimichurri Sauce 165
Peach Bourbon Barbecue Sauce 175
Remoulade 159
Satay Peanut Sauce 181
Spicy Tangy Barbecue Sauce 173
Tzatziki 169
Savory Roasted Nuts 209
seafood
   choosing fish 76
seasoning mixes
   Barbecue Rub 187
   Buffalo 186
   Herbes de Provence 185
   Jamaican Jerk 187
   Mediterranean 185
   Pumpkin Pie Spice 186
   Taco 188
serrano pepper 55
Sesame Ginger Vinaigrette 147
sesame seed oil
   Sesame Ginger Vinaigrette 147
shallots
   Citrus Vinaigrette 142
   Sesame Ginger Vinaigrette 147
   Tomato Balsamic Vinaigrette 147
shortcuts
   extras 37
shredded coconut
   Paleo Granola Bites 205
shrimp
   Lemongrass Shrimp 53
   Shrimp Louie 125
Shrimp Louie 125
sides
   Blanched Green Beans 105, 121
   Carrot & Apple Slaw 135
   Jamaican Rice & Peas 113
   Oven Roasted Potatoes 129
   Pickled Asian Veggies 55
   Pineapple Salsa 110
   Roasted Corn Salsa 71

Roasted Plantains 109
Sweet Potato Fries 131
Tostones 95
slaw
   Asian Slaw 51
   Carrot & Apple Slaw 135
   Mexican Slaw 101
   Southern Coleslaw 80
sleep 12
slowcooker
   Barbecue Pulled Pork 79
snacks
   Savory Roasted Nuts 209
soup 33
Southern Coleslaw 80
soy sauce
   Sesame Ginger Vinaigrette 147
spice mixes, See seasoning mixes
Spicy Tangy Barbecue Sauce 173
Spicy Tomato Jam 179
spinach 7
   Paleo Breakfast 43
sprouts 7
Steak Chimichurri 93
Steak & Sweet Potato 127
strawberries
   Strawberry Chia Pudding 199
   Strawberry Mojito Nice Cream 207
Strawberry Chia Pudding 199
Strawberry Mojito Nice Cream 207
stress 12
sweet potatoes
   Paleo Breakfast 43
   Sweet Potato Fries 131
Sweet Potato Fries 131
sweets
   Almond Bark 193
   Chai Latte Chia Pudding 195

T

tacos
   Barbecue Pulled Pork 79
   Mom-Style Taco 99
tamari
   Sesame Ginger Vinaigrette 147
tequila 75
Tequila Lime Fish 75
Tequila Lime Marinade 75
Teriyaki Chicken 57
Teriyaki Marinade 57
tomato
   Spicy Tomato Jam 179
Tomato Balsamic Vinaigrette 147
tomatoes
   Salsa Fresca 72
tomato paste
   Tomato Balsamic Vinaigrette 147
tools 63
   basic kitchen tools 63
   luxury kitchen tools 85
Tostones 95
turkey
   Mom-Style Taco 99
Tzatziki 169

V

vanilla bean
   Strawberry Chia Pudding 199
vegan adaptable
   All-American Burger 89
   Barbecue Pulled Pork 79
   Chicken Satay 61
   Chili Verde 65
   Lemongrass Shrimp 53
   Mom-Style Taco 99
   Steak Chimichurri 93
vegetables 6
veggies
   Pickled Asian Veggies 55
   Roasted Corn Salsa 71
vermicelli noodle bowls 53
vinaigrette
   Champagne Vinaigrette 142
   Citrus Vinaigrette 142
   Greek Vinaigrette 144
   Herbes de Provence Vinaigrette 144
   Mustard Vinaigrette 145
   Red Wine Vinaigrette 145
   Sesame Ginger Vinaigrette 147
   Tomato Balsamic Vinaigrette 147

W

white balsamic vinegar
   Mustard Vinaigrette 145

www.ingramcontent.com/pod-product-compliance
Lightning Source LLC
Chambersburg PA
CBHW061124070526
44584CB00033B/4211